OXFORD HANDBOOKS IN EMERGENCY MEDICINE
Series Editors   R. N. Illingworth, C. E. Robertson, and A. D. Redmond

D0947608

OXFORD HANDBOOKS IN EMERGENCY MEDICINE

This series has already established itself as the essential reference series for staff in A & E departments.

Each book begins with an introduction to the topic, including epidemiology where appropriate. The clinical presentation and the immediate practical management of common conditions are described in detail, enabling the casualty officer or nurse to deal with the problem on the spot. Where appropriate a specific course of action is recommended for each situation and alternatives discussed. Information is clearly laid out and easy to find — important for situations where swift action may be vital.

Details on when, how, and to whom to refer patients are covered, as well as the information required at referral, and what this information is used for. The management of the patient after referral to a specialist is also outlined.

The text of each book is supplemented with checklists, key points, clear diagrams illustrating practical procedures, and recommendations for further reading.

The Oxford Handbooks in Emergency Medicine are an invaluable resource for every member of the A & E team, written and edited by clinicians at the sharp end.

Psychiatric Emergencies

Stephen Merson
Consultant in Community Psychiatry
St Charles Hospital, London
and Honorary Senior Clinical Lecturer,
Academic Department of Community
Psychiatry, St Mary's Hospital Medical
School, London

and

David Baldwin
Senior Lecturer in Psychiatry
Faculty of Medicine
University of Southampton
and
Honorary Consultant Psychiatrist
Royal South Hants Hospital
Southampton

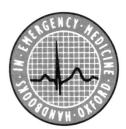

Oxford • New York • Melbourne
OXFORD UNIVERSITY PRESS
1995

Oxford University Press, Walton Street, Oxford OX2 6DP

Oxford   New York
Athens   Auckland   Bangkok   Bombay
Calcutta   Cape Town   Dar es Salaam   Delhi
Florence   Hong Kong   Istanbul   Karachi
Kuala Lumpur   Madras   Madrid   Melbourne
Mexico City   Nairobi   Paris   Singapore
Taipei   Tokyo   Toronto
and associated companies in
Berlin   Ibadan

Oxford is a trade mark of Oxford University Press

Published in the United States
by Oxford University Press Inc., New York

A catalogue record for this book is available from the British Library

Library of Congress Cataloging in Publication Data
Merson, Stephen.
Psychiatric emergencies/Stephen Merson and David Baldwin.
p. cm.—(Oxford handbooks in emergency medicine; v. 11)
Includes bibliographical references and index.
1. Psychiatric emergencies.   2. Crisis intervention (Psychiatry)
I. Baldwin, David, MB.   II. Title.   III. Series.
[DNLM: 1. Mental Disorders.   2. Emergencies.   3. Crisis
Intervention. WB 39 098 v. 11 1995]
RC480.6.M47   1995   616.89′025—dc20   94–49518 CIP
ISBN 019262478 4 (Hbk)
019262477 6 (Pbk)

Typeset by Footnote Graphics, Warminster, Wiltshire
Printed in Great Britain by
Biddles Ltd, Guildford & King's Lynn

Preface
(or how to use this book)

Psychiatric disorders are commonly encountered in general medical practice. This is so in the general hospital, both on the wards where it may coexist with physical disease, and in the casualty department where acutely ill patients may by-pass the normal pathways of referral. In primary care itself, up to 30 per cent of consultations have an important psychological component, although less frequently of an urgent nature.

This book is designed as a practical guide for those who are frequently required to manage patients presenting with acute psychiatric disorders. We are aware of the difficulties non-specialists often have in combining the formulation of the problem in diagnostic or other terms with the effective management of acute problems. We have therefore tried to avoid approaching the subject matter rigidly from the viewpoint of diagnostic classification. Instead, the format encourages the reader to obtain advice on practical management from the starting point of individual symptoms and syndromes which commonly occur in clinical practice. The chapter titles therefore clearly guide the reader to clinical problems.

The text is designed to take the reader through the steps of assessment, followed by management of the emergency to the stage where the problem is stable and consideration can be give to the planning of definitive treatment. We have avoided discussion of the later management and treatment of the important psychiatric conditions but make suggestions for further reading.

We hope this book will be of use not only to the casualty officer, the house officer, and the junior psychiatric trainee, but also perhaps to the more experienced but general medical practitioner, and those other than doctors working in the mental health field.

London   S.M.
January 1995   D.B.

Acknowledgements

The authors would like to thank Mary Pascal for her invaluable help with the typescript, and Peter Tyrer for his general encouragement. This book could not have been written without the support and forbearance of Shena Merson and Sally Baldwin to whom we wish to express our heartfelt thanks.

Contents

viii • **Contents**

PART 1

General principles of psychiatric emergencies

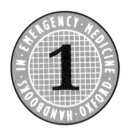

CHAPTER 1

History taking and the mental state examination

Introduction

- **Taking a history**   **Mental state examination**   **Physical examination**

The interview with a patient with psychological complaints has much in common with that of a patient with general medical complaints. Both involve an open discussion of the patient's current medical and personal difficulties, and both attempt to place these difficulties within a context allowing formulation of problems and potential solutions. Interviews with psychiatric patients, however, differ from other forms of medical assessment in two respects. First, the emphasis is naturally placed on emotional problems and social difficulties. Secondly, the process of interview and simultaneous examination of the patient's mental state amounts to an investigative and diagnostic tool in itself. Discussions with those who accompany the patient, and with those who are professionally involved in their care, are proportionately more informative in the assessment of the clinical problem.

Assessment of a patient who complains of psychological problems can, of course, be difficult. An assessment which is conducted in a thoughtful and empathic manner will allow the collection of relevant information, elucidation of any abnormalities of mental state, and the formulation of a provisional diagnosis. Most patients will find the process of interview beneficial, and a therapeutic alliance can be established between the patient and doctor, which will facilitate the subsequent plan of management.

Taking a history

Most of the patients who present with psychiatric problems to casualty departments or other emergency services are already known to the mental health services. This is especially true of those patients who present in a repetitive fashion, in or out of 'office hours'. Useful information as well as advice can therefore be obtained from those who are already in contact with the patient.

It should be possible for the hospital notes of a patient to be made available to the casualty department upon request, even at night and at weekends. Psychiatric medical records are often held separately from the notes recorded by other departments, and telephone calls with the 'duty psychiatrist' may be necessary before these notes are available. The introduction of computerized systems of record-keeping will allow, it is hoped, more access to this information in the future.

The information which is most relevant includes the diagnosis, the treatments (which the patient is or is meant to be receiving), and the identities of professionals involved as well as details of planned contacts. It should also be possible to establish whether the patient has a history of self-neglect, violence or suicidal behaviour.

The interview should be conducted in an appropriate and safe environment. Ideally, the interview room should be comfortable and private, and be equipped with a desk and stationery, a telephone, and an emergency alarm. The room should be slightly removed from the hurly-burly of the casualty waiting room, but easily accessible to patient and staff alike. Unfortunately, many of the rooms which are designated for the interview of psychiatric patients are inadequate or potentially hazardous. Such deficiencies should be drawn to the attention of the senior medical staff and relevant hospital administrators.

Most psychiatric patients can be safely seen on their own without the need for others to be present. It is prudent, however to inform the departmental staff whenever any decision is made to see a patient alone. It is foolish to see patients alone when the presenting problems include aggressive behaviour, or when the patient is known to have a history of violence. In these instances, or when the patient is irritable, hostile or demanding, or makes the examining doctor feel frightened, other staff should be present. Similarly, it makes sense to request the presence of others whenever a patient is accompanied by intimidating or demanding relatives or friends.

Many patients will be accompanied by friends, relatives, or those involved in their care. It is important to ensure that the accompanying persons remain in the vicinity whilst the interview proceeds—their premature departure can result in the loss of valuable information, may deny the patient emotional support, and can result in the patient being inappropriately abandoned with the resultant risk of unnecessary admission to hospital.

The interviewer should clearly introduce him or herself, and any others in attendance, and place the patient at ease. The doctor should sit between the patient and the door, within reach of an emergency alarm. The patient may wish for any accompanying persons to be present during the interview, although it is sometimes necessary to conduct an assessment of the patient alone. In these cases, the informants should be asked to remain in the department, and be made to feel confident that there will be an opportunity for discussion once the initial interview is complete.

The doctor should start by stating the purpose of the interview to the patient, and should tell him or her what is already known to the doctor. It is important to take reasonable control of the interview at the beginning, as otherwise a disjointed and potentially misleading assessment can occur. The patient should know the extent of time which is available, and should be told that the interview may involve a number of questions. They should be reassured that time will be made available at the end of the interview for discussion of any problems and the proposed plan of management.

Having established these external constraints to the interview, it is beneficial to proceed with an open question, which encourages the patient to start talking freely about his or her concern. The patient should be allowed to continue uninterrupted for a number of minutes, as this allows him or her to feel confident that their views are taken seriously. Often, the most valuable information is obtained during these first few minutes, which also allow observation of the patient's appearance and behaviour, and the detection of any abnormalities of speech such as increased pressure or incoherence. Having allowed the patient a certain degree of freedom, it is equally important to punctuate the discussion with statements clarifying the issues and ensuring they have been understood correctly.

It is not always possible to conduct an exhaustive assessment of every patient who presents to the Accident and Emergency department. Rather, it is important to obtain sufficient information to establish both the likely diagnosis and the possible consequences to the patient and others if the presenting problems were to be left unattended. The presenting psychological complaints should be clarified in some detail, together with the psychiatric and medical history. Specific enquiries should be made as to whether there is a history of suicidal behaviour, and current or previous alcohol and drug abuse. The social circumstances of the patient should be explored, including any planned contacts with professionals or impending Court appearances. If these items of information are not available from the patient, either because of an abnormal mental state or because of reluctance, it can be helpful to question those who accompanied the patient to hospital.

The majority of clinical information is obtained during the process of interview, rather than on examination. At the end of attempts to take a relevant history, the examining doctor should have a firm understanding of the nature of the presenting complaint, the details of any previous psychiatric history, and it should also be possible to harbour some suspicions regarding the nature of any underlying psychiatric disorder.

Mental state examination

Examination of the mental state in psychiatry is analogous to the physical examination in general medical or surgical practice. The symptoms which have been volunteered by the patient or elicited by the doctor are complemented by signs on examination which lead the doctor towards clinical syndromes and diagnosis. Casualty doctors are not expected to be expert in describing subtle abnormalities in psychopathology: it is important, however, for all doctors to be able to recognize significant signs such as the presence of marked disturbance of affect, thought disorder, delusional beliefs, abnormal perceptual phenomena or cognitive impairment. It is worth remembering that most psychiatric patients are familiar with the process of mental state examination, and will therefore be prepared for enquiries as to the presence or absence of abnormalities such as delusions of persecution or auditory hallucinations.

Typically, mental state examination proceeds from observations regarding the patient's appearance and behaviour, through a description of talk, affect, and thought, to perception, orientation, memory, and insight. This sequence can be altered as the interview and examination proceed, but it is worth developing a 'standard' format to make sure that nothing is missed. Particular enquiries should always be made regarding any suicidal thoughts, and a cognitive examination should always be performed.

Abnormalities of appearance or behaviour may suggest an underlying psychiatric disorder. For example, a patient dressed in a sombre fashion, with evidence of recent weight loss and self-neglect may be suffering from a depressive illness. Conversely, a brightly dressed or scantily clad patient may be experiencing a hypomanic or manic episode. The movements of a patient with depression are often slow and cumbersome, whereas manic patients are overactive, and may be disinhibited or overfamiliar. Observation of the patient should reveal any signs of movement disorder, attention being focused on the face for evidence of tardive dyskinesia, and on the limbs for signs of parkinsonism, akathisia or dystonia.

Similarly, abnormalities of a patient's speech may be suggestive of particular psychiatric disorders. Mutism is suggestive of schizophrenia or depressive stupor, whereas a loud and noisy patient, gabbling rapidly in an excited fashion may be suffering from mania. Typically, depressed patients exhibit soft, slow, and monotonous speech, with little spontaneity in conversation. Patients with schizophrenia may talk in a circumlocutory or incoherent fashion, or alternatively may demonstrate poverty of the content of speech, in which a limited number of items of speech are repeated without elaboration. It is useful to record verbatim any marked abnormalities of speech, as these are suggestive of thought disorder and underlying psychosis.

The patient's mood can be judged through observation of their manner and behaviour, but it is always important to make specific enquiries regarding low mood, anxiety, irritability, and elation. A patient's subjective account should be supplemented by an objective assessment of the prevailing affect at the time of their attendance in the department. Schizophrenic patients may show signs of affective blunting, in which the prevailing mood appears much the same throughout the interview, with a seeming loss of responsiveness to emotionally charged subjects. Conversely, certain patients with schizophrenia will demonstrate incongruity of affect, for example, describing the death of a loved one in a light-hearted and fatuous manner. Particular caution should be exercised when describing affect, as terms such as blunting or incongruity carry diagnostic significance.

Both the form and the content of the patient's thoughts should be determined. Abnormalities of the stream of thought include both the painful slowness of thinking of depressed patients with psychomotor retardation, and the exciting and stimulating flight of ideas characteristic of hypomania or mania. Abnormalities of the flow of thought include the giving of tangential replies to direct questions, loosening of associations, and 'derailment', these signs being suggestive of schizophrenia. Certain patients will describe abnormalities of the possession of thought, including thought insertion (in which the patient believes thoughts are placed into his or her head by external forces), thought withdrawal (the converse process whereby thoughts are believed to be extracted from the patient's thinking, against their will) and thought broadcast (a process akin to telepathy, in which patients believe that their thoughts are readily available to others in the immediate vicinity). These abnormalities when present in the absence of cognitive impairment are usually considered diagnostic of schizophrenia.

Examination of the content of thought may reveal signs of mental disorder, and will also allow an understanding of the patient's current preoccupations. Depressed patients will demonstrate excessive self-reproach or guilt, can report excessive concern regarding the presence of physical illness, and may be pessimistic for the future, with hopelessness or suicidal thoughts. Manic patients, by contrast, may regard themselves in an inappropriately esteemed fashion and may have unduly optimistic feelings regarding their future. Patients with paranoid disorders may indicate that they consider themselves to be the victim of plots or conspiracies. These abnormalities may be held with such intensity and fixity as to be delusional in nature. The presence of suicidal thoughts should always be determined, and if present the severity of suicidal intent can be calculated.

Major abnormalities of perception are suggestive of either 'functional' psychosis or 'organic' brain disease. Illusions are of little diagnostic significance, but specific enquiries should be made regarding the presence of hallucinatory phenomena, in each of the five sensory modes. Visual hallucinations without abnormalities in the other sensory modalities are strongly suggestive of intracerebral disease or toxic confusional states. Olfactory or gustatory hallucinations may be suggestive of complex partial seizures (temporal lobe epilepsy). It is important to develop a list of specific questions, with the aim of establishing whether or not hallucinations are present—for example, the question 'Have there been times recently when you have heard a noise or voice, without anyone being there?'

Most doctors, including many psychiatrists, tend to neglect the examination of the patient's cognitive function. Such an omission is both lamentable and potentially dangerous, as patients with 'organic' illness may be falsely regarded as suffering from 'functional' disorder, with possibly serious consequences. Examination of higher mental function includes testing the patient's attention and concentration, their orientation in time, place, and person, the registration of information, and the recall of both recent and distant memories. Abnormalities of the level of consciousness (for example, drowsiness or torpor) will preclude accurate assessment of these cognitive functions.

Typically, the process of interview itself reveals any signs of impaired attention or concentration. Mental state examination should include tests of attention, such as asking the patient to subtract the number 7 from 100 in a serial fashion, or to repeat the months of the year backwards. Significant abnormalities of attention may be suggestive of an acute confusional state or other intracerebral disease. Furthermore, impaired attention means that information obtained from the patient is likely to be unreliable, and particular caution should be exercised when formulating management plans.

Further assessment of cognitive function includes the testing of the registration of new information, and the recall of recent and distant memories. Registration can be assessed through asking the patient to memorize a five-item name and address, repeating it back to the examining doctor immediately. Recent memory can be assessed through asking the patient to recall the same name and address five minutes later. Distant memory is more difficult to assess, being individual in nature. It is common practice, however, for patients to be asked the dates of significant world events or recent items that have appeared in the newspapers. Impairment of short-term memory is unusual in the functional psychoses, and should always be considered to be indicative of the possible presence of organic brain disease.

The mental state examination traditionally ends with an assessment of the patient's insight. It is worth remembering that insight is probably a multi-dimensional phenomenon, and to ask questions accordingly. Certain patients, for example, may be prepared to accept that they are psychiatrically ill, but see no need for either care in hospital or treatment with medication. Other patients, by contrast, may wish to be admitted to hospital, but have no understanding of the change in their mental state or behaviour. Assessment of insight is of particular importance in psychiatric practice, as the most severely ill patients may resist any suggestion that it is appropriate for them to receive medical care and attention.

Physical examination

Although it could be argued that a full physical examination is necessary in all patients presenting to Accident and Emergency departments, there are certain situations where a physical assessment is probably unnecessary. It is sensible to ensure that a physical examination is performed in all 'new' patients, and in all other patients who may be well known to the service, but who may have presented with a new range of problems. Furthermore, it is advisable to perform an examination in all those patients who are known to have both a physical and psychiatric disorder. Elderly patients may be at particular risk of having a significant physical disorder missed. Finally, the presence of either an altered state of consciousness, or evidence of cognitive impairment on mental state examination should raise suspicion of intracerebral disease, and make physical examination mandatory.

The process of psychiatric interview and mental state examination can be difficult at first. The passage of time, and the development of clinical experience, will gradually ease any problem in assessing the mental health of patients. As in all other branches of medicine, it is essential to document any relevant findings within the medical notes, particularly the salient features within the history and any abnormalities on mental state examination. Notes should always contain some reference to the presence or absence of signs of significant depression, psychosis, or suicidal thoughts. Notes should be recorded in a legible fashion and be signed and dated clearly.

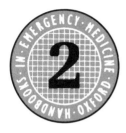

CHAPTER 2

General principles of psychiatric management

- Diagnosis Nosology Sources of information Variations
  in presentation Psychodynamic formulation
  Management Psychological treatment Drug
  treatment Notes Referral to Specialist Services

Diagnosis

As in other branches of medicine, management is naturally guided by diagnosis. Psychiatric diagnosis depends on the elucidation of descriptive psychopathology, and grouping of symptoms and signs leads logically to a medical diagnosis, in terms of a clinical syndrome, and potentially a more or less robust pathophysiological disease entity. This has the advantage of allowing the conversion of an apparently amorphous mass of confusing experiences and behaviour into a clear statement of opinion, which can thereby inform both communication with other professionals and management.

Nosology

The majority of psychiatric disorders are diagnosed solely on the basis of clinical features. This of course lays psychiatric diagnosis open to the charge of lacking validity and reliability, but it has also acted as a spur to the adoption of increasingly precise definition of symptoms and signs and their diagnostic significance (see below).

Systems of classification in current use share many features and every clinician likely to meet mentally ill patients in their work should have a working familiarity with these concepts. Serious psychiatric disorders are divided into those which are organically determined and those where no such organic aetiology is obvious. This of course is somewhat arbitrarily determined by the sensitivity of the tests employed to determine organicity, but is largely valid in clinical practice. Suspicion of an organic disorder should provoke more intensive investigation to elucidate a potentially treatable organic cause.

Functional disorders encompass a wide range of disorders which have traditionally been considered in two large groups: psychosis and neurosis. Both terms are now criticised for their non-specificity. The conventional distinction rests upon the accurate conception of reality by the patient, but it also includes a more general difference in severity.

The group of functional psychoses conventionally includes non-affective psychoses (including schizophrenia and related psychoses such as paranoid states) and affective psychoses (including the conditions of mania and depression). This distinction dates to the late nineteenth century and is generally accepted by most psychiatrists, despite the fact that some disorders stubbornly resist classification in this way.

The classification of the neuroses is widely held to remain unsatisfactory. These disorders include a range of features which are difficult to define adequately and tend to vary over time. Nevertheless traditional concepts such as obsessive-compulsive disorder, anxiety states, phobic disorders, and depressive disorders persist in the nosology alongside relative newcomers such as the eating disorders, somatoform disorders, and post-traumatic stress disorders.

Personality disorders remain controversial on the grounds that they are subjective and potentially pejorative. However, the concept of personality as a collection of recognizable and enduring character traits, and of its disorder in the sense of maladaptive behaviours leading to an individual's (or others') unhappiness is too well established in clinical practice to be readily discarded. It is increasingly regarded as an important factor determining the outcome of treatment in psychiatry, and is currently subject to considerable research attempting to improve its reliability.

Psychiatric systems of classification have weathered great changes over the last 20 years, but this has yielded dividends. For example, by reducing the numbers of clinical syndromes and by standardizing the criteria for their diagnosis the reliability (and validity) of diagnostic entities has been enhanced. These changes have also brought about a welcome convergence between the language of the research psychiatrist and of the clinician.

In addition, they have led to greater agreement in many respects between European psychiatrists (who use principally the International Classification of Disease of the WHO, currently in its tenth revision—ICD-10) and their North American counterparts loyal to the *Diagnostic and Statistical Manual of the American Psychiatric Association*, currently in its revised fourth edition (DSM-IVR). ICD-10 and DSM-IVR share more similarities than do their respective predecessors. They both avoid some of the perennial psychiatric controversies such as the concept of neurosis and the definition of syndromes on the basis of (often highly contentious) aetiological theories.

More importantly, both ICD-10 and DSM-IVR insist on explicit diagnostic criteria, usually involving the occurrence of a characteristic grouping of symptoms for a minimum duration and in the absence of other features pathognomonic of other disorders.

They have also both recognized the limitations of traditional psychiatric diagnosis in predicting prognosis and the response to different treatments. As a result both have begun to move towards a multi-axial system, which recognizes the importance of other dimensions such as social function, personality status, and physical health.

Sources of information

It is self-evident that the subject matter of psychiatry concerns abnormal behaviour. Behaviour itself may prevent psychiatric patients from conforming to interview, and can often demand assessments which depart from the conventional sequence of history followed by examination of the mental state. Patients all too often illustrate their behavioural disorder in their relationship with the professional whom they are consulting. Because a patient's history may be unreliable, other sources of information are of greater importance than in other branches of medicine. Neutral and knowledgeable informants should always be used to obtain descriptions of reportedly abnormal or uncharacteristic behaviour, and to shed light on the habitual or normal behaviour of a given individual.

Variations in presentation

Certain characteristics of patients may cause particular difficulties in the assessment of the mental state. The extremes of age, for example, are associated with variations in the presentation of several psychiatric disorders. Adolescents may present with disorders characteristic of childhood which differ from those of adulthood in many important ways and may best be viewed in the context of a family system. They are also prone to disorders more characteristic of adulthood, such as depressive illness or schizophrenia, and caution in reaching a diagnosis is therefore a virtue.

Some elderly patients with depressive disorders may present atypical features: with predominant somatic systems in the absence of clear disturbance of mood (masked depression); or with mood disturbance of anxiety or irritability in the absence of depression; or with little more than uncharacteristically histrionic behaviour. Another group of elderly patients may present the superficial appearance of cognitive impairment and only meticulous examination will reveal their 'pseudodementia' to be the result of the apathy, slowness, and inattention associated with depressive illness.

Those with mental handicap, whatever the aetiology, are more prone than the general population to all psychiatric disorders. In addition, the interpretation of reported symptoms and observed signs of mental illness is less reliable in those of low intelligence. Descriptions of experiences lack detail and may be rudimentary or simplistic. Accounts may be inconsistent on separate occasions and the individual easily led or suggestible.

Language is an obvious barrier to communication with patients from other countries. Less obvious cultural differences between patient and professional can produce more subtle obstacles to clear collaboration. Patients may be reticent as a result of concerns about family loyalty, cultural stigma attached to mental ill health, or contact with professionals of the other sex.

Additionally, the normal experiences of an individual from a different culture can be misinterpreted by professionals unfamiliar with this culture as a manifestation of mental illness. Unfamiliar religious or societal beliefs can appear to be strange and it is vital to seek the views of an informant who shares the culture of the patient before concluding that they are abnormal. Certain cultures, for example, those of the Indian subcontinent, recognize few linguistic terms to describe the mood state and rely on the description of bodily changes to express affective states, creating the possibility of misinterpretation.

Psychodynamic formulation

In addition to diagnosis, a psychodynamic formulation of the presenting problem can be attempted. This requires the professional to draw on sources of information about the patient other than direct self-report; it requires an awareness of the place of the patient in a system of relationships involving significant others, and an awareness of the relationship that is developing with attending professionals. An understanding of the patient's behaviour at this level is likely to lead to a more co-operative patient, as well as to a fuller understanding of their problem, even in an emergency situation.

This approach requires some familiarity with concepts such as transference (of emotions from elsewhere in the patient's experience to this relationship), and counter-transference, that is, emotions arising in the professional which can be understood as a reaction to subtle behaviours of the patient. Uncharacteristic emotions and impulses such as boredom, anger, impatience or desires to help beyond the boundaries of normal professionalism are likely to 'belong' in this way to the patient. It is important not to act on such impulses, but instead to consider them as clues to the internal world of the patient, taken in the light of what is known about the patient and their habitual way of behaving and relating to others.

Management

There are only a few psychiatric emergencies where a pause for a moment's reflection is impossible. These include active suicidal behaviour, and actively threatening and violent behaviour. In these situations the priority is to take control of the situation with clear instructions to colleagues regarding physical restraint and sedation if necessary.

One of the major decisions in the management of the acutely psychiatrically ill patient is the setting of their further management. Unlike medically ill patients, most psychiatric patients do not require to be nursed in a hospital bed as a result of physical debility. What they do require, particularly if they lack insight into their illness, is the physical presence of sympathetic others in a supervisory role. Management is likely to require the involvement of professionals if it includes medication, restraint in any form, or the planning and structuring of daily tasks. This can, however, be provided in a less restrictive setting than a hospital ward, for example, in the patient's home, a residential hostel or a day hospital. The possibility of management outside hospital should always be considered, but only in the light of the resources available to the patient.

Psychological treatment

In emergency work, treatment is likely to be predominantly 'physical' in nature: one of the contraindications for most psychological treatments is the presence of a crisis. However, the importance of clarity of explanation and reassurance of the patient should not be under-estimated.

Psychological treatments can be considered once the immediate emergency has passed. Patients vary considerably in their ability to use treatments such as cognitive–behavioural and insight-orientated psychotherapies: prerequisites are the commitment to a time-consuming and collaborative process, the ability to tolerate some delay before therapeutic gains can be made, and some facility to understand the theory underlying the particular method to be employed, as well as to engage in dispassionate self-reflection.

Drug treatment

When using physical treatments it is important to use the minimum effective dosage, to avoid polypharmacy and to monitor appropriately for adverse effects, taking into account the general physical condition of the patient and any coexisting medical condition.

Notes

As in other branches of medicine, documenting assessments and interventions is important, both from the point of view of verifying the clinical status of the patient and communicating this to colleagues, and for medico-legal purposes. Pay particular attention in this latter regard to documenting a patient's failure to follow medical advice, or reluctance to provide information when requested. Avoid pejorative statements or opinions that you would have difficulty defending. Try to stick to factual reports as far as possible. Be careful about confidentiality; in an era of multi-disciplinary working it is wise to have the explicit consent of the patient before sharing information with non-medical colleagues.

Referral to specialist services

It is always helpful for the receiver of a referral to know what the purpose of the referral is. This sounds obvious but research has shown that written referral letters between professionals fail to specify what is required and all too often the purpose of the referral is obscured by a poorly phrased request.

Before considering referral to psychiatric services, consider which question you are asking, and try to specify this in your referral. Legitimate reasons might include confirmation of your own assessment and clinical decision, advice on these same issues, a referral for the continuation of treatment, advice on the appropriate use of the Mental Health Act, or access to specific settings, including in-patient care, where psychiatrists are 'gate-keepers'.

PART 2

Clinical problems

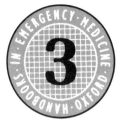

CHAPTER 3

Aggression

Introduction

- **Recognition   Interviewing   Management
  Drug Use**

Violence is a serious problem for those working in the health services. Casualty officers, working in the 'front line', are particularly vulnerable to acts of aggression, as are other workers in community settings. They may be expected to deal with hostile and agitated patients, but usually receive only minimal training in the techniques of preventing and controlling violence.

Recognition

Early recognition of the potential for a dangerous situation is the best way to avoid violence. Doctors and nurses should be able to identify those patients who are at particular risk of perpetrating violence. Although certain features (such as male sex, younger age, and alcohol intoxication) suggest an increased likelihood of aggression, the most important signs of impending violence are more immediate, and include increasing restlessness, hostility, verbal threats, and wilful damage to property.

   A number of psychiatric conditions are associated with increased risks of violence.

1. 'Organic' states:
   (a) acute confusional states;
   (b) alcohol intoxication;
   (c) alcohol withdrawal;
   (d) epilepsy.

2. Psychoses:
   (a) paranoid disorders;
   (b) mania.
3. Personality disorder;
   (a) explosive type;
   (b) antisocial type.

However, it is important to be aware that not all violence is associated with psychiatric disorder; violence may occur when a normal individual faces a situation of great tension and frustration. Patients who have recently been violent, or where police have been involved, should evoke more caution on the part of the interviewer.

Interviewing a potentially violent patient

Before the interview begins, attempt to obtain as much information from other sources as is possible, although without causing inordinate and frustrating delays. Locate the nearest 'panic button', and only proceed to assess the patient once you have established that other members of staff are in the immediate vicinity. Ensure that there is a clear exit away from the clinical area.

The interview room should be arranged so that the interviewer sits between the patient and the exit, preferably with some item of furniture, such as a desk, in between. Invite the patient to sit down or lie on an examination couch. Whilst taking a relevant history, stay at least an arm's distance away from the patient. Speak quietly, but loud enough to be heard, and avoid making sudden movements.

Conduct any physical examination steadily and purposefully, as any indecision or vacillation may make the patient more irritable. Avoid excessive eye contact, but do not turn your back to the patient. Exercise particular caution when taking blood samples, when it is sensible for needles and syringes to be removed promptly rather than left near the patient.

Management of actual or threatened violence

When interviewing a potentially violent patient it is important to allow the expression of the patient's grievances, and to listen attentively, but at the same time to avoid judgemental statements or to promise redress. This may allow the level of tension to diminish, particularly if the interviewer emanates an air of confidence and calm reasonableness.

When approached cautiously, calmly, and with common sense, most potentially aggressive patients can be managed effectively, and without violence. Occasionally, however, despite the use of precautions hazardous situations develop. In these circumstances, the first priority is the safety of the patient (through the prevention of self-harm), the safety of relatives, and of other patients and staff. The protection of property should be a relatively minor consideration.

When physical restraint is required, do not attempt any acts single-handedly, as this will probably result in personal injury and an escalation of violence. Ensure that other patients are escorted to a place of safety, and request the involvement of hospital security staff, and if necessary the police. Ideally, restraint should only be undertaken by staff who have received appropriate training in control and restraint techniques. Any action should be planned in advance, and the role of each person should be made clear. Attempts to restrain the patient should only be made when at least six members of staff are available—one for each limb and two for the body. One person should supervise, ensuring that an airway is maintained and that breathing is not restricted.

Pharmacological management of aggression

Many aggressive patients will need some form of sedative medication. When required, intramuscular preparations should be given while the patient is still physically restrained. Do not attempt to inject a patient who is not fully immobilized, as otherwise nursing staff may receive the injection inadvertently. Restraint should only be reduced after it has become clear that the situation is under control.

The underlying condition can then be clarified, and the appropriate management planned and implemented. Patients with acute alcohol withdrawal, for example, may require hospital admission, further sedation, and probable rehydration. Benzodiazepines can provide fairly rapid sedation, but repeated use is inadvisable in view of a reported potential for disinhibition and 'release' of further aggression. Neuroleptic drugs may have more sustained effects, especially when low to moderate doses are used repeatedly. Larger doses, prescribed on a one-off 'stat' basis, may wear off quickly or have unpredictable consequences. Neuroleptics possess epileptogenic properties, and should be used cautiously when the risk of seizures is high. Recently introduced oil-based preparations of neuroleptic drugs with a duration of action of 48–72 hours may avoid the necessity of repeated parenteral injections.

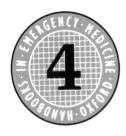

CHAPTER 4

Alcohol withdrawal and intoxication

Introduction

- **Delirium tremens   Hallucinosis   Wernicke's encephalopathy**

Chronic alcohol misuse is common in our society. This manifests in several ways which include physical ill-health, accidental injury, social dysfunction, crime, particularly of a violent nature, and behaviour (including, for example, suicidal behaviour) which may bring an individual to the attention of psychiatric services.

Services responsible for treating those with chronic alcohol related problems are several and may include primary care, the voluntary sector, and generic, and some specialist, psychiatric services. Multiple agencies can however be poorly co-ordinated with the consequent risks of duplication of services or, worse, absence of provision. Those working with psychiatric emergencies should ensure a working knowledge of the local availability of treatment services. The management of emergencies related to alcohol misuse is the main remit of this chapter.

Alcohol withdrawal syndrome (delirium tremens)

Delirium tremens ('DTs') is an acute confusional state that may complicate the withdrawal from habitual alcohol use, particularly in those who are alcohol-dependent. It is associated with a number of dangerous physical complications, and must be considered a medical emergency. However, with prompt recognition and adequate treatment, the prognosis is extremely good.

Recognition

Typically, delirium tremens occurs in the context of a recent reduction in the consumption of alcohol in an individual with a history of excessive or dependent use of alcohol. Difficulties in diagnosis include the non-specific nature of early symptoms (which may be similar to those in other psychiatric disorders), and the reluctance of many patients to report accurately their consumption of alcohol.

Common early symptoms of delirium tremens include intense anxiety, restlessness, and insomnia, together with physical symptoms such as tremor, tachycardia, fever, and ataxia. Other manifestations include perceptual disturbances such as illusions and hallucinations, which are typically fleeting or fragmentary in nature. Vivid and frightening hallucinations may lead to the development of transient, albeit firmly held, delusional beliefs. The clinical state may deteriorate rapidly to states of poor attention, disorientation, and confusion. The confusional states associated with delirium tremens have a characteristically sinister and intimidating tone, consistent with the content of the vivid hallucinations. Final stages of delirium tremens may include cerebral obtundity, coma, convulsions, and ultimately death.

Prevention

It is important to maintain a high index of suspicion that alcohol may be involved in any patient with acute anxiety symptoms. Signs of excessive or dependent use of alcohol, leading to an increased risk of delirium tremens include:

(1) round-the-clock drinking to avoid withdrawal symptoms;

(2) craving for alcohol;

(3) primacy of drinking over other activities;

(4) the development of tolerance.

Doctors should become familiar with the items within the CAGE questionnaire, and make rigorous enquiries regarding the consumption of alcohol when suspicion is raised. Remember that certain patients will be rendered unintentionally abstinent from alcohol as a result of extraneous circumstances, such as admission to hospital for the treatment of an unrelated medical condition.

Immediate management

This depends both on the stage to which the condition has progressed at the time of presentation, and on assessment of the likelihood of physical complications. Cases recognized early may be treated successfully outside hospital. Patients who are already in delirium, however, require full nursing attention to ensure adequate hydration and nutrition. Admission also provides reassurance and reorientation, and reduces the likelihood of accidental injury or confused wandering.

All patients with evidence of withdrawal symptoms require treatment with anxiolytic, sedative, and anticonvulsant drugs for periods of 7–14 days. Benzodiazepines combine all these properties, and can be given in a reducing regime of approximately 10–20 mg of diazepam (or equivalent) at 6 hourly intervals, reducing in a step-wise fashion, according to changes in the mental state. Patients in the early stages of withdrawal can be managed at home, providing they are not confused, are supervised by informal carers, and receive daily assessments over a period of 2 weeks. In patients with histories of convulsions, it is prudent to prescribe an anticonvulsant drug, such as phenytoin, in addition to benzodiazepine anxiolytics. When diet has been compromised, it is wise to prescribe vitamin supplements, in particular thiamine (vitamin B_1) to avoid the precipitation of acute encephalopathy. Thiamine can be administered either orally or by parenteral injection (intramuscular or intravenous administration).

Patients who are particularly frightened or bewildered may require considerable persuasion to remain in hospital, and it may be necessary to consider use of the Mental Health Act.

Alcoholic hallucinosis

Definition

Alcoholic hallucinosis is a relatively rare accompaniment of sudden fluctuations in the consumption of alcohol, usually on a background of pathological use. Typically, auditory hallucinations of a frightening and ghostly nature occur in the setting of clear consciousness over a period of 2–3 days. The relationship between this condition and delirium tremens is obscure.

Recognition

The sudden onset, clarity of perceptual disturbances, and history of a recent change in alcohol consumption distinguish alcoholic hallucinosis from the acute presentations of functional psychoses. Although the perceptual disturbances of alcoholic hallucinosis are qualitatively similar to those occurring in delirium tremens, hallucinosis is characterized by clear consciousness, which thereby distinguishes between these two conditions.

Immediate management

Reassurance and sedative anxiolytics, such as benzodiazepines, are generally all that is required until remission occurs spontaneously.

Wernicke's encephalopathy

Definition

Wernicke's encephalopathy is the clinical syndrome associated with acute thiamine (vitamin B_1) deficiency. The most common cause of thiamine depletion in the United Kingdom is chronic alcoholism, where the deficiency is largely a result of poor dietary intake. Other causes of thiamine deficiency include chronic gastrointestinal disease and malabsorption syndromes.

Recognition

The essential features of Wernicke's encephalopathy are an acute confusional state, nystagmus, ophthalmoplegia, ataxia, and polyneuropathy. Typically, the syndrome occurs in the context of chronic alcoholism, and is precipitated by exposure to a high carbohydrate diet, often during a period of improved nutrition as a result of treatment detoxification. High carbohydrate loads further deplete already deficient stores of thiamine, and may precipitate an acute encephalopathy.

Immediate management

The importance of early recognition cannot be overemphasized. Prompt treatment with parenteral thiamine will alleviate symptoms, and usually prevent progression to a chronic dysmnestic state (Korsakoff psychosis), which results from cell damage in the hippocampus and corpus mammillare. Many authorities recommend the routine use of thiamine supplements in those receiving treatment for alcohol detoxification.

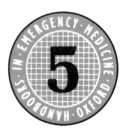

CHAPTER 5

Amnestic syndrome

Introduction

- **Recognition   Immediate Management**

Amnestic syndrome describes a well-circumscribed loss of short-term memory or ability to form and retain new information, occurring in the absence of impairment of other cognitive functions. Memory disturbance is often accompanied by other features of cognitive impairment, such as an alteration of conscious level, in cases of diffuse organic brain disease. It may, however, occur as a discrete abnormality, and it is for this syndrome that the term 'amnestic' is generally reserved. An amnestic syndrome should be considered to be the result of organic brain disease; psychogenic causes of amnesia are rare (see Chapter 13: Fugue).

Recognition

Presentation of amnestic patients will be determined by the speed of onset of the disorder. Those with an acute onset will complain of memory impairment, confusion or disorientation, or alternatively may be presented by family or friends concerned at amnesia for recent and current events. Amnesia of recent onset will often appear to be accompanied by an acute confusional state.

Amnesia of longer duration typically presents less as a direct result of changes in the cognitive state of the individual, but more often as a result of unanticipated changes in circumstances, which provoke social crisis of one sort or another. Typically, a dysmnesic patient may wander from his home, get lost and be unable to give an account of himself. The patient presents (by definition) as an unknown male or female unable to give a consistent explanation of recent events. The patient shows no features of a confusional state in the true sense (see Chapter 6: Confusion), and is usually able to speak coherently and cogently of biographical and other events remote in time.

Once suspected, formal testing of memory will readily reveal an impairment of the short-term recall of given information (such as a standard sentence or name and address) after 3 to 5 minutes during which time the subject is occupied with another intellectual task, such as simple mental arithmetic. Short-term recall can therefore be differentiated from the ability to reproduce material which is held within the span of attention. This may be accompanied by the description of increasingly unlikely and implausible ideas, in an attempt to explain the inconsistencies that emerge as the interview proceeds. This process is known as confabulation and may be mistaken for the delusional ideas of functional psychoses. In contrast to the short-term deficit of memory, there is relative preservation of the recollection of remote events, and procedural or complex acts are well maintained, thus differentiating the amnestic condition from acute and chronic confusional states.

Differentiation from other organic brain syndromes depends upon formal testing of the cognitive state of the patient, which may reveal other abnormalities such as agnosias, aphasias, or apraxias.

Amnestic syndromes are typically the result of bilateral, relatively well-circumscribed lesions in midline structures around the third ventricle, including the corpus mammillare and the medial dorsal thalamic nuclei. Causes of such lesions include:

(1) nutritional deficiency of thiamine (vitamin B_1) (Korsakoff psychosis associated with alcoholism or malabsorption syndromes);
(2) infective (encephalitic) causes, particularly herpes simplex encephalitis;
(3) trauma to the brain characteristically results in transient retrograde and anterograde amnesia. Localized lesions of

traumatic origin, however, can cause a discrete amnestic syndrome;

(4) post-ictal states usually include a significant element of disorientation and inattention, but amnesia may dominate the clinical picture.

Immediate management

The first priority of management is to exclude an acute confusional state and to ascertain the speed of onset. The history and mental state examination provide important information, but physical examination is mandatory, and investigations may be required particularly when a reliable informant is not available. These may include further neuropsychological investigations, a skull X-ray and possibly an EEG and CT brain scan. It is appropriate, if doubt remains, to admit the patient to hospital and observe the mental state over a period whilst investigations can proceed.

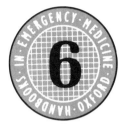

CHAPTER 6

Confusion

Introduction

- **Recognition   Immediate management**

The descriptive term 'confusion' is so frequently used among medical and lay persons as to have largely lost its specific meaning. Partial impairment of consciousness (with features such as disorientation, disturbance of memory, abnormal perceptions and false beliefs) is better described as an 'acute confusional state' thus distinguishing the clinical condition from popular experience. Although often used synonymously with 'confusion', 'delirium' is a particular form of acute organic brain syndrome, characterized by a rapid onset, fluctuating course, and brief duration. Perceptual disturbances are common and motor activity disturbed.

Recognition

Doctors are rather poor at recognizing acute confusional states in their patients, frequently misdiagnosing such problems as dementia or functional psychoses.

The cardinal features of acute confusional states include:

(1) alteration of consciousness, ranging from overarousal and excitement, to drowsiness and torpor;
(2) impairment of attention, registration, and recall;
(3) disorientation in time and place—disorientation in person is rather less frequent.

These features vary with the course of the illness, and are typically worse at night.

Additional features may include:

(1) behaviour ranging from overactivity and aggression to retardation and mutism;
(2) repetitive and manneristic rituals;
(3) affective disturbance, including elation, fear, depression, irritability, and changeability of mood;
(4) slow, muddled or disordered and inconsequential thinking;
(5) delusions, particularly of a persecutory nature;
(6) abnormal perceptions, including misinterpretations of the surrounding, and hallucinations.

It is vital to distinguish between organic and functional causes of acute behavioural disturbances. Illusions, visual, tactile or olfactory hallucinations, and profound disorientation are strongly suggestive of an organic disorder. Features such as ataxia, dysarthria, and incontinence are uncommon manifestations of functional psychosis.

Immediate management

The first task in the management of acute confusional states in patients in a concise and accurate assessment of the mental state. The next step involves elucidation of the underlying physical cause. The more common causes of acute confusional states include the following, all of which are more likely to induce confusion in the elderly and those with pre-existing organic brain disease:

(1) prescribed medication, including analgesics, anticholinergics, digoxin, and cimetidine;
(2) drugs of abuse, including barbiturates and benzodiazepines;
(3) alcohol withdrawal;
(4) infection, particularly with accompanying septicaemia;
(5) metabolic disorders, such as electrolyte disturbances and the complications of diabetes;
(6) organ failure—cardiac, respiratory, renal or hepatic;
(7) Intracranial causes, including head injury, subdural haematoma, encephalitis, and post-ictal states.

It is apparent, therefore, that when faced with a 'confused' patient, simple physical examination, including elementary measures such as taking the patient's temperature, listening to the chest, and feeling for a full bladder, may allow a causative factor to be determined and appropriate management instituted. Occasionally, however, exhaustive investigations may fail to reveal any identifiable abnormality.

Treatment of any underlying cause is the cornerstone of management. Symptomatic relief may be required, to alleviate subjective distress, and to prevent disruptive or intrusive behaviour and wandering. The patient should be nursed by familiar staff in a well-lit but quiet room. Attempt to explain to the patient what is occurring, even though he or she may appear oblivious to your activities. Repeatedly orient the patient in time and place, and constantly remind him of your identity.

Try to restrict the prescription of drugs, and certainly avoid polypharmacy. Occasionally, sedatives may be used for the daytime relief of agitation and distress (preferably without causing excessive drowsiness), and the night-time induction of sleep. Drugs, when used, should be employed at low dosage and for as short a time as possible.

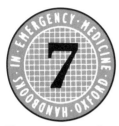

CHAPTER 7

Deliberate self-harm

Introduction

- **Initial assessment   Suicide intent scales   Immediate management**

Assessment of the risk of suicide is one of the most common problems in emergency psychiatry. An appropriate level of enquiry into suicidal thinking should be undertaken for all patients with psychiatric disorder or psychological complaints. For those who have presented following acts of deliberate self-harm, evaluation must be especially systematic and thorough, and management planned appropriately.

The incidence of deliberate self-harm (of which approximately 90 per cent of cases involve self-poisoning) now accounts for around 20 per cent of admissions to general medical wards and is the most frequent reason for admission to hospital in young female patients. The increasing number of cases of deliberate self-harm has led to a recent change in suggested guidelines, so that automatic referral to a psychiatrist is no longer considered to be feasible, or mandatory. Rather, all doctors should be acquainted with the factors indicative of suicide risk, and become familiar with the management strategies employed by local specialist services. This is supported by the fact that, given suitable training, doctors and nurses without formal psychiatric experience can be as effective in detecting patients at high risk of completed suicide as specialist mental health professionals.

Initial assessment

It is important to remember that deliberate self-harm is not a single clinical entity, but rather the final common pathway from a range of motivations, difficulties, and disorders.

Assessment of suicide risk after deliberate self-harm should be performed in surroundings that are conducive to a frank discussion of personal problems. Curtained spaces within an Accident and Emergency department are far from ideal—the relative seclusion and privacy within modern short-stay wards is preferable. An interview should only be attempted once the patient is medically fit, but conversely should not be delayed unnecessarily, as patients may develop unrealistic rationalizations of any problems during the interim period. It is sometimes difficult to obtain a reliable history when interviewing patients who have harmed themselves. Problems may arise through embarrassment, in either the patient or the doctor. Many individuals will be reluctant to discuss personal feelings and may actively resist attempts at understanding. A patient's mental state may fluctuate widely following a suicide attempt, and 'snapshot' assessments can have little predictive validity. Many who harm themselves are isolated or living in conflict with others, and the lack of objective information from relatives or friends may hamper accurate assessment.

The following schedule is recommended in the assessment of suicide risk:

(1) attempt to establish an adequate rapport. Be aware of any negative feelings evoked in professionals by those who self-harm, and expressions by the patient of hostility and resentment;

(2) gain some understanding of the event and circumstances of the few days prior to the suicide attempt. In particular, try to judge the amount of preparation and concealment, the true intention, and whether the outcome was affected by unforeseen eventuality;

(3) explore any personal or social circumstances which present difficulty to the patient, and construct a problem-orientated formulation;

(4) obtain an alcohol history;

(5) perform a brief psychiatric history and mental state examination;

(6) refer to specialist services when appropriate.

The risk of completed suicide in those who have committed acts of deliberate self-harm has been the subject of considerable research. A range of scales has been developed, and include those items which predict an increased risk of suicidal behaviour. Regrettably, such scales have little predictive power on an individual basis, as personal characteristics and circumstances change with time. Those who do eventually commit suicide would typically have been considered at risk of suicide prior to their death. However, many who would be considered at risk do not harm themselves again. If scales are the sole means by which 'at risk' patients are identified, many more patients will be followed up than is either indicated or necessary.

Suicide intent scales

Suicide intent scales, however, have some use in reminding doctors of the questions that are necessary when making an assessment of patients seen after acts of deliberate self-harm. Beck (1974) developed a scale with the following items:

1. Preparation:
   (a) act planned in advance;
   (b) suicide note written;
   (c) action in anticipation of death, for example, writing a will.

2. Circumstances of the act:
   (a) patient was alone;
   (b) timed such that intervention would be unlikely;
   (c) precautions taken against discovery.

3. Sequelae of the act;
   (a) did not seek help;
   (b) stated wish to die;
   (c) stated belief that the act would have proven fatal;
   (d) sorry the act failed.

An alternative approach is to see how clearly the patient approximates the 'stereotype' of a completed suicide. The closer the fit, the greater the long-term risk of suicide. Completed suicide is associated with male sex, older age, single status, and social isolation. A history of previous deliberate self-harm, affective disorder, alcohol misuse or serious medical illness is often found in those who kill themselves. The risk of suicide is increased by a factor of 100 compared to that in the general population when there is both a recent history of deliberate self-harm and persistent, distressing suicidal ideation.

Although psychological problems are common in patients who have attempted to take their lives, formal psychiatric disorders are rather rare. This is a fact that often inspires disbelief, but nevertheless experience will reveal it to be true. Motivations underlying deliberate self-harm are often complex or fleeting. Deliberate self-harm is not necessarily determined by the presence of a mental disorder. Certain patients may wish to die, whereas others may be ambivalent, caring little whether they survive or succumb. Many individuals have been hurt by friends or partners, and others may wish to express their anger through self-harm. It is not uncommon for patients to describe an unbearable sense of tension, relieved by suicidal behaviour. Others may wish simply to escape briefly from difficult circumstances. Simple craving for attention is rather uncommon.

Depressive disorders account for the majority of cases of deliberate self-harm in which there is a definable mental disorder. Major depression and recurrent brief depression (RBD) are both characterized by low mood, agitation, pessimism, and suicidal thoughts. In these patients, the findings of delusional ideas of guilt of worthlessness, or the presence of continued suicidal intent, markedly unpleasant mood states or derogatory mocking or instructive hallucinations must all be considered to increase the risk of completed suicide. The sheer unpredictability that is characteristic of RBD may be an especially destabilizing factor, impelling patients toward reckless and punitive actions. Alcohol dependence and personality disorder are common in completed suicide victims. Schizophrenia is recorded rather infrequently, but the risk of suicide in psychotic patients who have harmed themselves is especially hard to determine, and the threshold for admission to hospital in these circumstances should be low.

Immediate management

Clearly, subsequent steps in management are determined by the findings at interview and on examination. Five issues require consideration:

(1) the risk of suicide, both in the short and longer term;
(2) the need for psychiatric treatment;
(3) the type of treatment which may be required;
(4) the location and supplier of treatment;
(5) alternative approaches, when psychiatric help is unnecessary.

The main concern of casualty officers should be in ascertaining the risk of suicide. Specialist services should be responsible for the other endeavours.

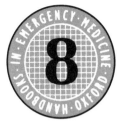

CHAPTER 8

Delusions

Introduction

- **Recognition   Immediate management   Admission to hospital   Treatment**

The concept of delusion is one of the most important in psychiatry and is intimately connected with the notion of psychosis. Psychotic disorders tend to be those with the most serious consequences for the patient and his or her family. Delusions are defined as pathological forms of false beliefs; their importance in psychotic illnesses lies in their propensity to displace the usual beliefs of individuals, which are subject to confirmation or refutation by the evidence of our perceptions. They may then lead to behaviour which is both uncharacteristic of the individual and incomprehensible to the observer.

Many mentally healthy individuals are prone to mistaken and erroneous assumptions, and therefore falsity in itself is not sufficient to imply that a belief is delusional. Several criteria need to be met before a belief can be confidently assumed to be delusional. Delusions must preoccupy an individual, to the extent of virtually excluding other thoughts. They are held with unwavering conviction, and are resistant to reasoned contradiction. Delusions have personal significance, and are not understandable in terms of personal or cultural origin.

Delusions should be distinguished from two related phenomena: overvalued ideas and partial delusions. Overvalued ideas are preoccupying notions that dominate an individual's thinking, but which lack the intense personal involvement and sense of complete conviction that characterize delusional beliefs. An example would be the insistence on the significance of a scientific discovery by an individual that is not shared by his peers in the scientific fraternity. Partial delusions are beliefs which an individual may recognize as being potentially false, and usually represent delusional ideas that are either emerging with illness or resolving through treatment. An example would be the expression by an individual that she is being unfairly harassed by the police whilst at the same time accepting that she may be mistaken and being prepared to consult a psychiatrist.

Not all delusional beliefs are inherently unlikely or bizarre. Patients may even still be considered as deluded when the belief they hold is factually correct. This apparent contradiction occurs when a conviction is founded upon incorrect reasoning or interpretation of evidence. Thus a patient may be (rightly) convinced that his wife is unfaithful to him, not on the basis of objectively reliable evidence, but on the basis that a hallucinated voice informs him that this is the case, or that he mistakenly reads this significance into his neighbours cheerful greeting to him in the morning. Thus the formation of a delusion involves not just a false belief, but also a process of morbid interpretation of evidence.

It can sometimes be difficult to differentiate delusional beliefs from other beliefs which we accept as normal. Religious conviction and original scientific concepts are examples. Either may approach the borderline of delusional belief if the content becomes excessively idiosyncratic.

The content of delusions varies very widely. This can form the basis for a typology of delusional beliefs which has diagnostic utility, since certain delusions are characteristic of particular psychiatric disorders. Thus grandiose delusions involving belief in special physical or spiritual powers or a privileged status are characteristic of mania. Conversely the delusions of psychotically depressed patients are typically guilty, hopeless, self-blaming, and hypochondriacal, and in their ultimate expression (the nihilistic delusion) deny the individual's very existence. Delusions of persecution are common to both affective and non-affective psychoses and therefore lack diagnostic specificity: however, depressed patients typically accept their persecution as their just desserts, whereas the reaction of those with mania or paranoid psychoses is likely to include resentment and outrage.

Many sorts of delusion occur in schizophrenia, but some are regarded as pathognomonic of the disorder: these have in common the failure to identify thoughts and emotions as belonging to the self and the attribution of their origin to external agencies. Experiences such as the reception of alien thoughts into the individual's mind or of outside control of one's actions are examples of such passivity experiences.

Other specific delusions may so dominate the mental state as to justify the description of the disorders accordingly, some of which have received eponymous titles. Some of the more common are:

- Morbid jealousy
- Erotomania (de Clerambault's syndrome), involving delusions of loving by one of high rank
- Delusions of replacement by doubles (Capgras syndrome)
- Monosymptomatic hypochondriacal psychosis, involving delusions of parasitosis, disease, or bodily change (dysmorphophobia).

Delusions are important abnormal mental phenomena, as they are restricted to the more serious psychiatric disorders. Delusional beliefs may result in irresponsible and uncharacteristic behaviour, ranging from self-neglect to antisocial confrontation or dangerous and life-threatening activity. Delusions are also associated with significant impairment of social and occupational roles. Finally, the presence of delusions influences the insight of a patient into his or her illness, and may therefore affect their readiness to engage in treatment.

Recognition

Patients with delusions may present in a variety of ways, depending on the nature and content of the delusional belief.

Persecutory (paranoid) delusions

Persecutory delusions typically dominate the mental life of an individual, and may cause the patient to seek help directly.

The victim of perceived persecution may seek redress through legal channels, and be referred to psychiatric teams, if liaison between the services is particularly close. Occasionally, the patient may refer him or herself to a doctor having implicitly recognized the true nature of his or her problem. More typically, however, the patient will be presented to doctors by concerned relatives or neighbours, discomforted by odd or puzzling behaviour.

Grandiose delusions

Patients with grandiose delusions, which often occur in the setting of excitement, euphoria, and disinhibition, often present following conflict with other people who do not share the patient's beliefs. The police may become involved, when a grandiose individual fails to recognize the consequences of their disturbed behaviour.

Depressive delusions

Depressive delusions typically occur in the context of depressive illness. Typically, they have a hypochondriacal, self-reproachful or pessimistic quality. Persecutory delusions may occur in which case the depressed patient is usually not outraged or angry, but rather accepts persecution as a deserved punishment. Because of the prevailing sense of apathy, psychotically depressed patients are unlikely to present themselves for treatment, but will be reluctantly brought to attention by worried friends and relatives.

The presence of delusions is established through examination of the content of speech and thought expressed by a patient. It is rather uncommon for patients to describe their delusional beliefs in a forthcoming manner. Persecuted patients are suspicious and mistrustful, depressed patients apathetic and fatalistic, and manic individuals distractible and impatient. Systematic enquiry related to beliefs is therefore a necessary routine. Patients' behaviour may provide an indication of the nature of their preoccupying thoughts, and useful information can be obtained from those who have witnessed any changes in behaviour if the informants know the patient well. It is important to ensure that delusions are indeed false before the patient is identified as mentally ill. Sometimes even the most bizarre claims turn out to be true.

Immediate management

Treatment of a deluded patient should aim to reduce the intensity of abnormal preoccupations, such that more appropriate mental activity can regain its rightful place. This should have the simultaneous effect of reducing uncharacteristic disruptive or dangerous behaviour.

The first step in management is to establish a relationship of mutual trust. Arguing with a deluded patient in a logical fashion is a waste of time. Such endeavours only encourage the patient to mistrust the doctor, and will lead to the breakdown of any therapeutic alliance. Rather, it is preferable to guide the interview into areas where there is a reasonable chance of finding agreement. For example, whilst avoiding arguing with a patient who believes him or herself to be pursued by vindicative enemies, it may be fruitful to ask him or her what effect such a perceived persecution is having. Even the most deluded patient may be helped by such an approach. Most psychiatrists draw little from psychodynamic theory during the definitive treatment of delusions. Psychotherapeutic techniques, such as the interpretation of unconscious material and the transference of emotions, have little utility in the management of someone who is unable to distinguish between reality and fantasy. Although the presence or absence of delusional beliefs governs steps in management, the content of delusional thoughts should never be neglected. Understanding of the nature of such thoughts permits entry into the patient's inner world, and guides decisions regarding the safety of the patient and others.

When patients are willing to accept treatment, it is sensible to monitor compliance and to maintain reassurance and encouragement. This can be provided in a psychiatric unit, but many patients will benefit from domiciliary care, particularly when relatives are present and frequent visits can be made by mental health professionals. In certain cases, however, informal treatment is not possible, and a decision has to be made as to whether the patient can be allowed to continue suffering through his or her delusions, or whether it is appropriate to compel admission to hospital through the use of the Mental Health Act.

Admission to hospital is likely when delusional thoughts render behaviour dangerous, either to the patient, or to those in the vicinity. Delusions of persecution, for example, may lead an individual to take the law into his or her own hands, particularly when the patient feels him or herself to be the subject of abuse or ridicule. Depressive delusions of guilt or terminal illness may lead to suicidal thoughts and behaviour. Delusions of deformity in a child may lead the mother towards catastrophic action. The passivity delusions of schizophrenia can result in unpredictable acts of any kind.

The risk of an individual acting on the basis of delusional beliefs is subject to a number of modifying factors. For example, knowledge of how the individual has reacted in similar circumstances may allow a reasonable prediction of the likelihood of self-harm or aggression. Conversely, intoxication with alcohol may lower the threshold for the expression of violent impulses. A patient who lives in a sympathetic and supportive family may not act upon erroneous conclusions, whereas one who is exposed to a critical atmosphere may feel impelled towards violence.

Compulsory admission to hospital

Concern about the risk of violence should lead to admission to hospital immediately under the provisions of Section 2 of the 1983 Mental Health Act. If a delay in obtaining the two medical recommendations which are necessary for such a Section would entail some risk to life or limb, it is appropriate to arrange admission under the provisions of Section 4. This requires only a single medical recommendation, but allows admissions for only 72 hours. During this time, a second opinion can be sought. When health is jeopardized, continuing avoidance of treatment may be sufficient cause for admission to hospital. Self-neglect, malnutrition, and increasing destitution may represent grounds for admission. In such cases it is important to consider not only the patient's mental health, but also the likelihood of a response to treatment. When health is deteriorating, and treatment readily available, it is appropriate to consider admission under the provisions of Section 3 of the Mental Health Act, as this will allow treatment for a period of up to 6 months.

Treatment of delusions

Psychological approaches have only a limited role in the treatment of delusions, particularly in acutely unwell patients. The presence of delusions is a contraindication to the use of insight-orientated psychotherapy, as the patient finds difficulty in separating metaphor from reality. Cognitive styles of psychotherapy have begun to be researched, but only in the treatment of chronic and well-circumscribed delusions. Acute treatment of the deluded patient, therefore, is principally reliant on the use of antipsychotic medication. With treatment, the intensity of delusions typically diminishes within a few weeks, although changes in behaviour may be noticeable rather earlier. It is important to ensure continuing compliance with treatment once beneficial changes in mental state occur, as early withdrawal of medication usually leads to relapse.

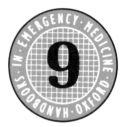

CHAPTER 9

Depression

Introduction

- **Variations in presentation   Increasing recognition
Immediate management   Risk of suicide   Referral**

Depression is a common and disabling disorder. Although estimates vary, it seems that approximately 20 per cent of women and 10 per cent of men will suffer from depression at some time during their lives. Community surveys indicate that 3–6 per cent of adults are suffering from depression at any one time.

Although common, depression can be difficult to recognize. The majority of depressed patients probably present to their general practitioner but are also very prevalent in general hospital settings, including Accident and Emergency. Difficulties in the recognition of depression result from a reluctance to discuss emotional problems, the presentation of physical complaints, and the limited time that is available for consultations in primary care settings. It is likely that in addition to many depressed individuals who fail to seek help, another substantial group do present to their doctors but are not recognized as suffering from depression. Even when patients are diagnosed as depressed, the treatment which they receive may be insufficient or may prove ineffective as a result of poor compliance with treatment.

Recognition

The most classic form of depression is one known as 'melancholia'. This disorder has a number of characteristic features, including low or unpleasantly changed mood, a pervasive loss of interests (anhedonia) and suicidal thoughts. Melancholia is often accompanied by the so-called 'biological symptoms' of depression that include:

- early morning wakening;
- diurnal variation of mood (feeling worse in the morning);
- weight loss;
- loss of memory;
- constipation;
- loss of energy.

Examination of melancholic patients may reveal signs of self-neglect. Movements may be retarded, with avoidance of eye contact and a loss of expressive gestures. Speech may be soft, slow, and monotonous. Few thoughts appear to enter the patient's mind, and those that do are depressive in nature, with the self being regarded as worthless, life meaningless, and the future without hope. Suicidal thoughts are common and may be difficult to resist.

The majority of depressed patients, however, do not exhibit the classical features of melancholia. Symptoms can be milder and more variable. Typical forms of depression are characterized by low but reactive mood, psychological and somatic features of anxiety, an increased preoccupation with presumed physical ill-health, and low self-esteem. 'Biological' symptoms may be absent or even be reversed, with increased appetite and weight, and hypersomnia (sleeping excessively). The symptoms and signs of anxiety may seem to dominate the clinical picture, but close questioning will reveal the underlying features of depression.

Psychiatrists probably see a rather unrepresentative sample of the most severely depressed patients. The definitions of depression which are derived from samples of psychiatric inpatients may have less relevance in general hospital or primary care settings, where many depressed individuals will not fulfil the accepted criteria for major depression, because their illness is too mild, too short, too long, or without social consequences. Arguably, the two forms of depression that are of the most relevance to general practitioners are 'depressive episode' (ICD-10, F32), and 'mixed anxiety and depressive disorder' (ICD-10, F41.2). The typical clinical features of these disorders are detailed in Tables 9.1 and 9.2.

Many experts have argued that anxiety can be distinguished from depression on the basis of differences in symptoms and signs, the course of illness, and response to treatment. However, it has become increasingly clear that the two conditions have a considerable overlap. These observations have led the World Health Organization to include a category of mixed anxiety depression within the ICD-10. Patients who fulfil the diagnostic criteria for 'mixed anxiety and depressive disorder', have symptoms of both anxiety and depression, with neither set of symptoms being sufficiently severe to justify a separate diagnosis (see Table 9.2).

Variations in the presentation of depression

A small proportion of depressed patients suffer from a psychotic illness. They may consider themselves to be wicked or guilty, believe that a terminal illness is present, or maintain that they are destitute. Some will expect to receive punishment for their supposed misdemeanours. These beliefs are usually found to be groundless and delusional. Certain patients may hear voices which tell them that death is imminent, or instruct them to commit suicide. Insight is often impaired, with the patient being unable to appreciate the severity of their illness and the need for treatment.

Table 9.1 • Depressive episode (ICD-10, F32)

Typical symptoms
Depressed mood
Loss of interest and enjoyment
Reduced energy

Other symptoms
Reduced concentration and attention
Reduced self-esteem and self-confidence
Ideas of guilt and worthlessness
Bleak and pessimistic views of the future
Ideas of self-harm or suicide
Disturbed sleep
Diminished appetite

Table 9.2 • Mixed anxiety and depressive disorder (ICD-10, F41.2)

- Symptoms of both anxiety and depression.
- Neither set of symptoms sufficiently severe to justify a separate diagnosis.
- When both syndromes are severe enough to justify individual diagnoses, both disorders should be recorded and the category should not be used.
- If symptoms occur in close association with significant life changes or stress, the category of adjustment disorder should be used.
- Excludes persistent anxiety depression (dysthymia).

Elderly patients may have unusual variants of depression. Cotard's syndrome is a rare form of psychotic depression in which the patient holds the nihilistic belief that part of his body is diseased and rotting, or that death is either imminent or indeed has already occurred. In depressive pseudodementia, patients may complain of forgetfulness, and examination may reveal signs of poor attention, disorientation, and limited registration and recall of new information. Only when the underlying depression is sought and treated is the cognitive impairment found to have been a secondary phenomenon.

Depressed mood is common in children but its diagnostic significance is often unclear. The symptoms of childhood depression vary with age, with abdominal pain and changed behaviour being prominent in young children, and guilt and suicidal thoughts rather more common in adolescence. When compared to adults, it seems that depressed children are more frequently troubled by hallucinations, but are less commonly afflicted by delusional ideas.

Increasing the recognition of depression

Although a few patients may present with unequivocal, obvious symptoms and signs of depression, such situations are relatively uncommon. In practice it is often difficult to recognize the depressed patient. Detection may be a little easier if certain strategies are employed by the examining doctor:

- Become conversant with the common clinical features of depression, such as low mood, disturbed sleep, altered appetite, and impaired concentration.

- Enquire into the presence of psychological symptoms when patients present with somatic complaints that have no apparent 'physical' cause.
- Suggest further discussions of the patient's problems with their family doctor if insufficient time is available.
- Suspect depression in certain situations, for example:
  - the 'thick folder' patient;
  - those with chronic physical illness or social adversity;
  - problem drinking of recent onset;
  - reports of changed behaviour in children and adolescents;
  - complaints of memory loss in the elderly.
- Take steps to determine the severity of illness before attempting to ascribe it to any cause: the presence of precipitating factors does not obviate the need for further assessment and treatment.

Immediate management

Treatment of acute depressive episodes

No two clinical situations are identical: the following is simply a broad guideline for the management of acute episodes of depressive illness:

- Establish the presence of a depressive disorder.
- Exclude underlying severe mental disorders such as schizophrenia and dementia.
- Determine the severity of depression:
  - psychotic illness: refer to psychiatrist;
  - severe depression: refer to psychiatrist;
  - moderate illness: will probably benefit from an antidepressant drug;
  - mild depression: counselling may be appropriate.
- Establish whether other illnesses are present:
  - cardiovascular disease, glaucoma, and prostatism are relative contraindications for certain tricyclic antidepressants;
  - patients with hepatic or renal disease or epilepsy may benefit from referral to a psychiatrist for advice on selection of an antidepressant.

- Choose an antidepressant drug that is known to be clinically effective, reasonably well tolerated, and relatively safe in overdose;
- Inform the patient that although side-effects of antidepressant drugs are apparent from the beginning of treatment, beneficial effects have a delay in onset of 2–3 weeks;
- Prescribe at low dose for 1–2 days and then increase to a dose which is known to be effective.

The risk of suicide in depressed patients

Suicidal thoughts are an integral part of depressive illness, and all depressed patients must be considered to be at risk of self-harm. Approximately 15 per cent of those with a diagnosis of recurrent affective disorder will eventually commit suicide. Accurate identification of patients at particular risk is not easy, but the following demographic and clinical variables are suggestive of an increased risk of suicide:

- Older age (although the incidence of suicide in younger people is increasing).
- Male sex.
- Single status (especially if recently single, for example, following divorce or bereavement).
- Physical illness (for example, chronic obstructive airways disease or epilepsy).
- History of aggressive behaviour.
- Presence of coexisting personality disorder or alcohol abuse.
- Particular types of depressive disorder, such as psychotic illness or recurrent brief depression.

However, the overwhelming factors to be considered in assessing suicidal risk are the following, and either of these two features may increase the risk 100-fold.

- **Recent** history of suicide attempt (even if relatively trivial at first sight).
- **Current** admission by the patient to having suicidal thoughts.

If enquiry about suicidal thoughts produced ambiguous or uninformative answers, the patient may be asked if they are hopeless about the future, or whether they have feelings of desperation or a feeling that they must do something drastic about their situation. Suicidal patients are likely to respond positively to both of these points.

Referral of depressed patients to a psychiatrist

Referrals to the psychiatric services are influenced by a number of factors, including the clinical features of the patient, pressure from external sources (for example, relatives or friends), the experience of the examining doctor, and the availability and competence of the specialist facilities.

Referral to a psychiatrist may be appropriate in the following clinical situations.

- When the diagnosis is uncertain, for example in elderly patients or those with chronic physical illness.
- Psychotic illness (that is, depression characterized by the presence of delusions, hallucinations or loss of insight).
- Severe depression (for example, patients with marked loss of appetite or weight, or those showing profound psycho-motor retardation).
- Depressed patients who have made a recent suicide attempt.
- Patients with distressing or intrusive suicidal thoughts or those troubled by feelings of hopelessness or despair.
- Failure to respond to an adequate course of antidepressant medication.
- When specialist treatments are necessary (for example, adjuvant medication, cognitive therapy or ECT).

In the absence of these particular problems, it is appropriate for the patient to be managed, at least at first, by their general practitioner.

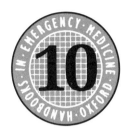

CHAPTER 10

The 'disorganization syndrome'

Introduction

- **Recognition   Immediate management**

The 'disorganization syndrome' is a term used to encompass a group of relatively non-specific features which are associated with psychotic illness, particularly schizophrenia. These include disturbance of mood (including lability and incongruity of affect and perplexity) to disorder of the form of thought (disrupted stream or association of thoughts, and opaque or impoverished thinking) and abnormal behaviour (odd, socially inappropriate, or inconsequential behaviour). This concept corresponds broadly to the earlier concept of hebephrenic schizophrenia whose integrity as a sub-syndrome of schizophrenia with particularly poor response to treatment is increasingly recognized by psychiatrists. This syndrome often co-exists with symptoms of other sub-syndromes of schizophrenia in the same patient.

Recognition

Typically, such patients are presented by others: family and friends, or sometimes the general public, the police or other public services, concerned at an individual's failure to give a coherent account of seemingly purposeless and neglectful behaviour. This may range from behaviour provoking puzzlement to that inconveniencing or alarming others. This may have emerged either because the patient has chronic symptoms and has escaped from a social environment which had hitherto contained and tolerated his eccentricities (often an after-care hostel) or because his symptoms have recently deteriorated.

Disorder of the form of thought is often prominent. Psychiatrists talk of disorder of the form of thought to describe observable abnormalities of language in its role in the symbolic representation of concepts, as opposed to abnormalities of production of the motor act of speech, such as dysarthria and dysphasia. Formal thought disorder usually involves abnormalities of the semantics of language, though errors of syntax are evident in more florid forms. Semantic difficulties may include some of the following processes:

• confused use of metaphor and synonym;
• spurious associations, for example rhyming or alliteration;
• idiosyncratic new words (neologism);
• loosening of meaningful associations between ideas.

The disorganization syndrome is easily mistaken for other psychiatric disorders unless careful examination of the mental state is made. For example, the inconsequential fatuousness and silly facetiousness can be mistaken for hypomania. The apparent inattention, incomprehensibility or poverty of speech and purposeless behaviour may resemble the features of a confusional state, or indeed a frontal lobe syndrome, with which it shares many similarities.

The absence of any reliable history necessitates the interview of an informant to confidently reach a diagnosis. In its absence a period of observation of behaviour in a psychiatric ward is usually sufficient.

Immediate management

The aim of treatment is to ascertain the diagnosis, and to prevent danger or exploitation (particularly of a sexual or financial nature). Subsequently, it is necessary to arrange a suitable setting for further physical treatments, initially in the form of reinstatement of lapsed antipsychotic treatment, but perhaps leading to behavioural management over a longer period.

If a history of known psychosis is not forthcoming, admission to an acute psychiatric ward is indicated for further observation, investigation, and treatment. Administration of antipsychotic drugs may rapidly alleviate perplexity and thought disorder, and thereby allow a more lucid communication and description of the mental state, aiding further management decisions.

CHAPTER 11

Drug withdrawal and intoxication

Introduction

- **Withdrawal syndromes   Intoxication   Psychosis management   Notification of drug dependence**

Drug misuse is rather more common than is popularly imagined. The consumption of illicit drugs, such as diamorphine (heroin) or cocaine, is not restricted to youth. Use and abuse of analgesics and hypnotic drugs is common in more senior members of the community. Doctors see only a minority of drug misusers: most drug use is recreational, dependence being relatively infrequent. Certainly, only a small minority of drug abusers come into contact with the psychiatric services, and those who do have more psychological, social, and physical problems than the majority who fail to come to medical attention.

Drug-related problems are therefore common, and result in frequent presentations to Accident and Emergency departments, particularly in inner cities. It is important to adopt a non-judgemental attitude to drug abusers, as paternalistic or condescending approaches may simply act to maintain the patient's problems. Doctors should be concerned with minimizing potential damage, both to the patient, and to society.

Drug misuse is associated with a wide range of problems:

(1) physical problems, include withdrawal syndromes and the complications of drug misuse such as abscess formation, septicaemia, endocarditis, and infection with hepatitis B or HIV viruses;

(2) psychological complications including anxiety, depression, suicidal behaviour, aggression, and psychosis;

(3) social difficulties which arise from the priority given
to the supply of drugs by misusers, including financial
burdens, unemployment, homelessness, and problems
in forming and maintaining relationships. Drug habits
may be supported by prostitution and illegal activity.

Typically, drug misusers present to Accident and Emergency
departments at times of crisis. Patients may present as a
result of drug withdrawal, or following an accidental or
deliberate overdose. Intoxication with drugs is not an uncommon presenting problem, but instances of 'bad trips' and
drug-induced psychosis are rather less frequent.

Drug misusers are often destitute and desperate. Many
resort to challenging behaviour when presenting for medical
help. Certain patients may resort to deception, such as the
simulation of physical illness, or may lie with respect to
personal details. Others may be importunate, seductive or
confrontational. Theft of prescription pads and headed note-
paper is a recognized problem, as is the disappearance of
medical equipment, including needles, swabs, and syringes.
A supportive approach is therefore best combined with an
element of extra vigilance.

Withdrawal syndromes

Most withdrawal syndromes are characterized by a combination of psychological and physical problems. Many of the
psychological difficulties are rather non-specific, but somatic
symptoms and signs aid diagnosis. Opiate withdrawal, for
instance, is associated with marked agitation, apprehensiveness, and fearfulness, which steadily increase in severity
over a period of 48 hours. Physical symptoms include
nausea, abdominal, and musculo-skeletal cramping, examination revealing signs of shivering, mydriasis, lacrimation,
rhinorrhoea, and sweating. Although unpleasant, opiate
withdrawal is not especially severe, resolving without last-
ing ill-effects in the majority of cases.

Barbiturate withdrawal, by contrast, is a serious and
potentially life-threatening medical emergency. The syn-

drome is rather similar to delirium tremens complicating alcohol withdrawal. Young people may present when their illicit supply of barbiturates is interrupted, older patients when their legal but therapeutically antiquated prescription of barbiturate hypnotics is no longer renewed. Acute confusional states are not uncommon, and the risk of epileptiform seizures is high. Patients should be admitted to hospital and stabilized medically, oral doses of phenobarbitone elixir being prescribed on a regular basis until the patient is comfortable and alert.

The existence of a true benzodiazepine withdrawal syndrome is still somewhat controversial. A substantial minority of chronic benzodiazepine users experience difficulty when drugs are stopped, or the dosage reduced. Many of the features of a putative withdrawal syndrome are similar to those of the condition for which the drug was prescribed. Certain authors have argued that a particular constellation of symptoms (including paraesthesia, tinnitus, vertigo, and hyperacusis) is pathognomonic of the withdrawal from benzodiazepines. Rarely, acute confusional states or seizures may occur. Although distressing, most of the symptoms which arise after stopping benzodiazepines are not especially severe, and it is sensible to regard a patient who presents to casualty demanding an immediate prescription with some suspicion.

Intoxication with drugs

Drug intoxication is probably the most common psychiatric syndrome seen in drug abusers presenting to Accident and Emergency departments. Intoxication with alcohol is a familiar clinical entity. Solvent abuse is widespread amongst adolescents, particularly those living in socially deprived areas. Clinical features of intoxication with solvents include agitation, restlessness or drowsiness, glazed or fixed expression, slurred speech, and clumsy gait. Habitual glue sniffers may develop a characteristic rash in the perioral region. Heavy intoxication may prove fatal, through asphyxia, cardiac dysrhythmia or personal injury.

Abuse of phencyclidine ('Angel Dust') is more prevalent in the United States than in Europe. Typically, intoxication is characterized by apparent drunkenness, or by 'eyes open coma', in which an alert patient is mute and unresponsive to painful stimuli. Agitation, when present, can be marked, and behaviour most disturbed. Aggression and suicidal behaviour are not uncommon. Intoxication with phencyclidine constitutes a psychiatric emergency, and hospital admission is invariably required.

Drug-induced psychosis

Persistent use of certain illicit drugs may be linked to the development of psychotic illnesses that are in many respects indistinguishable from other forms of mental illness, such as schizophrenia. Indeed, the similarities between amphetamine psychosis and schizophrenia contributed to the dopamine hypothesis of the aetiology of schizophrenia.

The clinical features of drug-induced psychosis are as variable as those seen in other forms of serious mental disorder. Amphetamine psychosis is characterized by stereotypic and manneristic behaviour, perseveration, instability of mood, persecutory delusions, and a variety of abnormal perceptual phenomena, most especially visual hallucinations. In rare cases, there may be features suggestive of an organic brain syndrome, including impaired attention, defects in registration and recall, and disorientation.

The psychotic illness associated with prolonged use of cocaine bears certain similarities to the above picture. Affective instability, however, is even more marked and tactile hallucinations ('cocaine bugs') are commonly described. Cannabis misuse may be associated with acute relapse in chronic schizophrenia, but there is no consensus as to whether cannabis itself can produce a psychotic illness. Prolonged consumption of cannabis is, however, occasionally associated with the development of an 'amotivational' syndrome, similar in many ways to the negative features of schizophrenia.

The similarities between drug-induced psychosis and

schizophrenia may render distinction between the two diffi-cult. Factors which are suggestive of a drug-induced origin include:

(1) recent and abrupt onset in young patients;
(2) previous history of alcohol or drug abuse;
(3) physical signs of drug misuse, such as needle puncture marks, thrombosed veins, and damage to the nasal septum.

The initial management of drug-induced psychosis is the same as that for psychoses arising from other causes. A urine sample should be obtained as soon as possible, so that a screen for metabolites of commonly abused substances can be performed. Preferably, patients should be observed and managed without recourse to psychotropic medication. In practice, however, the severity of many drug-induced states is such that treatment with neuroleptic drugs is required.

Strategies employed in the management of drug dependence

Traditionally, two approaches have been used in the man-agement of drug dependence. The first, based on moral argu-ments, was aimed at enforcing abstinence. The second, adopting a medical approach, is that drug dependence is an illness, which warrants and requires medical attention. More recently, however, a third approach has been utilized, largely as a result of the HIV pandemic. This approach con-siders that HIV is a greater danger to individual patients and society as a whole than drug misuse is in itself. 'Harm reduc-tion' therefore, aims to minimize the spread of HIV through the provision of safe and reliable sources of drugs and drug-taking equipment.

The approach which is adopted locally is the concern of the drug dependency specialist services. Casualty officers should become familiar with local arrangements, and adhere to agreed policies. It is worth remembering that there is no reason to give a prescription of drugs of dependence to unknown 'addicts' presenting to Accident and Emergency departments.

Notification of drug dependence

A doctor is obliged to notify the Chief Medical Officer in writing of any person that is considered to be addicted to one or more of a range of drugs (see Table 11.1).

Table 11.1 • 'Notifiable' drugs of dependence

Cocaine	Methadone
Dextromoramide	Morphine
Diamorphine	Opium
Dipipanone	Oxycodone
Hydrocodone	Pethidine
Hydromorphine	Phenazocine
Levorphanol	Piritramide

The notification forms that are in common use require completion of personal details such as the name and address, sex and date of birth of the patient, together with the date of first attendance, the names of drugs that are being abused, and a statement as to whether or not the patient is receiving a prescription of medication.

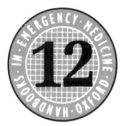

CHAPTER 12

Fear and panic

Introduction

- **Recognition   Immediate management**

The stresses and strains of everyday life are often accompanied by apprehension and feelings of tension, which are usually appropriate and may indeed be beneficial. The performance of challenging tasks may be facilitated by increased levels of arousal and attention. At other times, however, anxious feelings arise from nowhere, or seem to be out of proportion to circumstances. Anxiety should then be regarded as a pathological rather than an understandable phenomenon. As such it is a common and relatively non-specific symptom of many psychiatric disorders.

Anxiety symptoms may also occur in patients with disorders of personality which render them liable to cope poorly at times of adversity. It is, however, difficult to diagnose personality disorder on the basis of a single interview, as careful evaluation of many aspects of functioning is required, and access to an informant is desirable.

Recognition

Anxiety is characterized by both psychological and physiological features:

1. Psychological symptoms and signs include apprehensiveness, unfounded worrying, fearfulness, inner restlessness, irritability, and exaggerated startle response.
2. Physiological features can be regarded as either:
   (a) autonomic in origin, with features such as palpitation, breathlessness, epigastric discomfort, diarrhoea, and urinary frequency; or

(b) musculo-skeletal, problems including muscular tension, stiffness, and tremor.

A significant proportion of anxious patients develop panic attacks. Typically, such attacks represent recurrent bursts of severe anxiety which are not restricted to particular situations or sets of circumstances. Attacks are of sudden onset, brief but severe, and seemingly unpredictable. Patients may present in crisis, disabled by palpitations, marked breathlessness, fainting, and profuse sweating. Many believe that death is imminent, or at the very best they will remain alive but completely lose control and 'go mad'. Patients who have experienced recurrent panic attacks over many months may develop an anticipatory anxiety, in which there is reluctance to be alone or in public places. Fear of panicking itself may induce further panic attacks.

Immediate management

Diagnosis of an anxiety state should only occur when more serious underlying disorders, both physical and psychiatric, have been excluded. Physical conditions which may be complicated by anxiety include cardiac disease (for example, supraventricular tachycardia), thyrotoxicosis, hypoglycaemia, and phaeochromocytoma. Psychiatric illnesses, such as schizophrenia, bipolar affective disorder, and depressive illness, may all be characterized by anxiety, the true nature of the underlying disorder only being revealed when close questioning and thorough mental state examination reveal the presence of specific and pathogonomic symptoms. Panic attacks are uncommon in those aged over 65 years, where especially careful assessment is therefore required. Similarly, the diagnosis of anxiety should be questioned when patients of a previous equable temperament present in crisis, without evidence of undue stress.

A variety of techniques have been used in the acute management of patients with panic attacks. Hyperventilation results in distressing physical symptoms (such as paraesthesiae and muscular spasm), which anxious patients interpret as being indicative of underlying physical illness. Control of breathing is therefore essential. Doctors and nurses should instruct patients to take slow and measured breaths and note how symptoms and signs fade as breathlessness diminishes. Occasionally, patients may benefit from breathing in and out of a paper bag for a few minutes, but this manoeuvre should only be used when cardio-respiratory causes of anxiety have been excluded.

Clearly, the treatment of anxiety arising from underlying illness is dependent on the nature of the primary condition. Patients with primary anxiety states may benefit from a range of treatments, including pharmacological approaches and cognitive-behavioural therapies. Definitive treatments such as these should be instituted by either general practitioners, or specialist psychiatric services. Casualty officers should avoid requests for medication by anxious patients. Acquiescence to patients' demands will serve merely to reinforce dependence and further compromise coping skills.

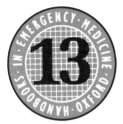

CHAPTER 13

Fugue

Introduction

- **Recognition   Immediate management**

Fugue is an uncommon syndrome, characterized by wandering away from the usual environment accompanied by the simultaneous loss of memory. It may have either psychogenic or organic causes. Psychogenic causes are probably rather more common, but organic disease is occasionally implicated.

Recognition

Typically, the subject in fugue is brought to the attention of medical or other public services by concerned members of the general public after having been unable to give an adequate account of him or herself. In extreme cases, the affected individual may have moved away from home, adopted a new and radically different personal identity, and lived as such for several weeks. More commonly, however, fugue states are characterized by the loss of only certain aspects of memory, and by a rather limited wandering from the usual surroundings. When interviewed by medical or nursing staff, the patient may have no presenting complaints, but often reports that he or she is lost, or may state that he or she has not knowledge of the events of the recent past. Examination may reveal evidence of self-neglect and of a recently itinerant existence. The patient may appear dehydrated, but evidence of malnutrition is rare. Observable testing of memory will usually reveal relatively well-circumscribed defects of registration and recall. In cases of fugue associated with organic disease, however, there may be additional signs of poor attention, and of more wide-spread cognitive impairment.

Immediate management

Management of the patient in fugue should be conducted in a sensitive manner. Naturally, the first task in management is to attempt to distinguish organic and psychogenic causes of fugue, although this may prove difficult. Full interview and physical examination is mandatary and a thorough mental state examination with evaluation of cognitive function is required. As much information as is possible should be obtained from other sources—from informants where available, and from careful scrutiny of any documents and articles that the patient may possess.

Psychogenic causes of fugue include:

(1) depressive illness;
(2) dissociative states;
(3) malingering.

Fugue has traditionally been considered to be precipitated by severe stressful events, such as the termination of an intimate relationship or the threat of an impending court appearance. It has been argued that in these cases, fugue is a form of hysterical condition, with primary and secondary gains for the patient. More recent reports, however, describe the prevalence of depressive syndromes in patients with fugue, and prolonged wandering may indeed be a suicide 'equivalent' in some patients. Sensitive enquiries into the presence of suicidal thoughts or feelings of despair should therefore always be made.

In contrast to the goal-directed wandering that is typical of psychogenic fugue, organic factors may produce a rather more erratic and less purposeful picture. The wandering that may be a complication of complex partial seizures (temporal lobe epilepsy, for example), is usually purposeless, and it is also uncommon for a new identity to be assumed with this condition. In organic fugue, conversation is likely to be limited and fragmented, and physical examination may reveal evidence of neurological abnormalities.

The more common physical causes of fugue include:

(1) head injury;
(2) epilepsy;
(3) intoxication with alcohol.

Most cases of fugue are brief, typically resolving within a few days. Recovery is usually abrupt and complete. Nevertheless, it is appropriate to arrange the admission of the patient to hospital, to ensure personal safety and continuing health. Whilst in hospital enquiries regarding the patients origin and difficulties can be made. Underlying causes should be sought, and treated where appropriate. Rehydration and dietary measures may be required in those who have wandered without concern for their welfare.

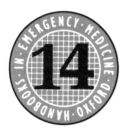

CHAPTER 14

Hallucinations and other perceptual disturbances

Introduction

- **Recognition   Immediate management**

Hallucinations and other abnormalities of perception are important features of many of the more serious psychiatric disorders. The perception of a stimulus can be conceptualized as involving two stages. Energy of a particular form (for example, sound or light) acting on a receptor organ causes the generation of a neurochemical signal, which is relayed to cortical sensory areas that record the crude sensation. The subsequent transmission of this image to cortical association centres results in the interpretation of this image in the context of other inputs to the organism as a whole.

Hallucinations are a form of false perception. They are sensory percepts (as opposed to sensations) which lack corresponding and causative stimuli. Hallucinations are beyond voluntary control, and occur in objective space alongside other verifiably true perceptions. Hallucinations may occur in any of the five sensory modalities, but are most commonly encountered in the visual and auditory spheres.

Their importance is twofold. First, hallucinations can be distressing. This is particularly so when occurring for the first time, when the experience can be disorienting, perplexing or frightening. The content of hallucinations may be so unpleasant as to provoke vigorous and sometimes dangerous attempts at avoidance. Secondly, the occurrence of hallucinations may often precede or provoke the onset of delusional ideas, which can themselves lead to serious behavioural consequences.

Recognition

Hallucinations require differentiation from other perceptual abnormalities. Prominent amongst these are misperceptions (also called illusions), which are inaccurate interpretations of correctly sensed information. A variety of factors may influence the interpretation of a correctly sensed event, including the prevailing mood state, the degree of attentiveness, and the context against which the perception occurs. An anxious patient may interpret a subjective sensation of tachycardia as indicative of cardiac disease, and a delirious patient his shadow as a potential assailant.

Hallucinations should also be distinguished from other perceptual experiences which are less associated with psychosis:

(1) sensory distortions, where one aspect of a real object (for example, its shape, size, colour or sound) is altered;

(2) pseudo-hallucinations, a form of voluntary mental imagery which are distinguished from 'true' hallucinations by a perceived origin within the of the subject's body ('subjective space') and by their voluntary nature. Pseudo-hallucinations may be a feature of non-psychotic depressive illness and certain forms of personality disorder (such as the emotionally unstable or borderline category);

(3) agnosia, that is, the inability to recognize a correctly sensed object usually associated with cerebral dysfunction;

(4) derealization and depersonalization, where perception of the surroundings and oneself becomes altered in the presence of an abnormal mood state, typically one of severe anxiety;

(5) several types of perceptions not indicative of mental illness, including eidetic images (voluntary recall of a remembered image), retinal after-images, and pareidolia (images provoked by abstract sensory impressions, such as seeing faces in a glowing fire).

Hallucinations themselves are not necessarily indicative of mental illness. They are known to occur in normal individuals during the transitional states of altered consciousness between waking and sleeping (hypnopompic and hypnagogic hallucinations, respectively). Furthermore, true hallucinations may accompany intoxication with a variety of hallucinogenic drugs, including LSD, Ecstasy/MDMA, cocaine, amphetamine, and cannabis.

Hallucinations may occur in any of the five senses. The sensory modality is diagnostically of some guidance: for example, auditory and visual hallucinations are more characteristic of functional psychoses, whereas hallucinations in the other modalities (gustatory, olfactory or tactile) should raise the possibility of an organic cause such as temporal lobe epilepsy. Hallucinations in organic psychoses may be brief, fragmentary or episodic, and are often 'elemental' (that is, unsophisticated images, such as simple sounds, or coloured shapes or lights with no obvious significance to the patient). This contrasts with the more elaborate, and sustained hallucinations which are commonly found in the functional psychoses.

Other features of hallucinations may provide some clues to the underlying diagnosis. Hallucinations that are mood congruent, for example, gloomy, frightening, and apocalyptic where the mood is depressed, or inspirational or ecstatic when the mood is euphoric, support the diagnosis of affective psychosis. Mood-congruent auditory hallucinations often speak in the second person in an insulting or adulatory manner to the patient, and often provoke uncharacteristic behaviour as a result. Mood-incongruent hallucinations, where the content of the hallucination is at odds with the prevailing affect of the patient, are associated with non-affective psychoses, particularly schizophrenia. Mood-incongruent auditory hallucinations typically refer to the individual in the third person, often commenting on their actions or repeating their thoughts aloud.

Immediate management

The immediate objectives of management are:

1. Relief of distress due to intrusive and unpleasant hallucinations. Effective management of a hallucinated patient

depends on their insight and ability to co-operate within a therapeutic alliance. Explanation that a patient's experiences are understood, that he is safe and can be helped are not always sufficient to guarantee co-operation. A calm and supportive environment (e.g. a side room or a psychiatric ward) can be helpful. Orally administered antipsychotic drugs may begin to reduce the intensity and intrusiveness of hallucinations within hours, but their effect may not be noticeable until some days have passed. Hallucinations occurring in organic states may be made worse by antipsychotics, and consideration should be given to treatment with anticonvulsants, but only after thorough investigations.

2. Avoidance of irresponsible or potentially dangerous behaviour. This requires an assessment of the degree of danger. Distress provoked by frightening or unpleasant hallucinations may lead to self-harm. It is important to be aware that patients with complete insight into the morbid nature of a hallucination may nevertheless be so distressed by it as to be driven to self-harm as a means of relief.

   More critically, dangerous actions can occur in response to hallucinated commands, and reports that voices are urging suicide or assault should always be taken seriously. Insight is one factor in predicting the likelihood of a response to a hallucinated command, but others are also important. Some will protect the individual from suicidal behaviour (such as religious belief in the sinfulness of suicide, or concern at the likely distress to loved ones). By contrast, violence to the self or others is more likely to occur in an individual with a history of impulsive behaviour, or after the ingestion of alcohol or other disinhibiting drugs.

3. Restoration of normal mental activity, including mood, volition and beliefs, free of influence from hallucinations. In the short term this will require the administration of antipsychotic drugs. Relief from abnormal perceptual phenomena is likely to be associated with a simultaneous reduction in the intensity of delusional beliefs, and beneficial effects on affect, judgement, and behaviour.

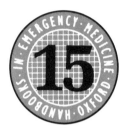

CHAPTER 15

Mania and hypomania

Introduction

- **Recognition   Immediate management   Treatment of mania and hypomania**

Hypomania is the term used to describe a syndrome involving sustained and pathological elevation of mood, accompanied by other changes in function such as disturbances of physical energy, sleep, and appetite. Mania is a similar syndrome, in which the individual additionally holds delusional ideas (i.e. is psychotic). Bipolar affective disorder (manic-depressive psychosis) is an episodic illness, where periods of normal psychological functioning are interrupted at intervals by periods of either mania or depression.

Mania and hypomania occur less frequently than other functional psychoses. They are however associated with high levels of morbidity, mortality, and social impairment. Mania and hypomania may be complicated by violence or other behavioural disorders, and account for a significant number of involuntary admissions to hospital (i.e. admissions under the Mental Health Act 1983).

Despite this the prognosis is very favourable with a likelihood of remission of symptoms, though of course recurrence is a recognized feature of these disorders. The syndrome of hypomania may sometimes occur as a manifestation of other underlying psychiatric illnesses, such as schizoaffective psychosis or schizophrenia.

Recognition

The essential feature of these disorders is a persistent elevation of mood. As in all affective disorders, it is important to establish (usually with the aid of an informant) that the observable mood state is not within the normal range for that individual. Other features of hypomania or mania include:

(1) ideas of an unrealistic or grandiose nature (to a delusional degree in mania);
(2) an increased range and tempo of thought;
(3) motor over-activity (the subjective experience of increased stamina, and observable agitation);
(4) diminished need for sleep;
(5) increased interests in socialization, food, and sex;
(6) irritability;
(7) distractibility.

The mood changes associated with these conditions are often complex, and at times difficult to recognize. This is because increased lability of mood is as characteristic as elation or euphoria. Mood may be fluctuant, oscillating between bonhomie, hostility, irritability, anxiety, worry, and gloom. Such rampant fluctuation of mood is characteristic of a sub-group of bipolar patients with so-called mixed affective states or rapid-cycling illness. It is sometimes difficult to distinguish between an anxious and agitated depressed patient, and a hypomanic individual who worries and frets. Abnormal thoughts may include not only grandiose ideas, but also other mood-congruent ideas such as self-reference and persecution. Differentiation from cases of schizophrenia may be difficult, particularly when such thoughts are accompanied by excitement and over-activity. Similarly, the mood lability of mania or hypomania may be mistaken for the fatuous euphoria of hebephrenic schizophrenia.

Immediate management
Recognition of a problem and acceptance of treatment

Typically, manic illnesses are characterized by poor judgement and reduced insight. The manic patient is unable to equate his or her elevated mood, enhanced energy, and brimming self-confidence with ill health, and can see no need for help or treatment. The patient's assessment of any situation tends to be overly optimistic, and poor decisions regarding treatment are common. Participation in any discussion is limited through the distraction caused by a constant pressure of bubbling and exciting ideas.

When dealing with manic patients, it is worth remembering that the mood state may be brittle and labile. Congenial good humour can quickly turn to irritability and anger in the face of minor degrees of frustration. The manic patient is often humorous and disinhibited, and can enthuse others with their excessive confidence. This is beguiling and attractive, and good spirits are often contagious. However, this can also lead to errors of judgement by doctors, and it is wise to err on the side of caution when making management decisions.

Management of a manic patient outside hospital is only possible when the patient is sufficiently insightful to comply with treatment, and where there is considerable and dependable informal support. Admission to hospital is therefore indicated in the majority of cases.

Prevention of disturbance

The behaviour of a manic patient may be impulsive, capricious, over-confident, ill-considered, and irresponsible. It can lead to over-spending, sexual promiscuity, and illegal acts. Disinhibited behaviour may threaten relationships, employment, livelihood, and reputation. Furthermore, manic patients may act without regard for personal safety or health, and may neglect their nutrition to the point of exhaustion.

When planning treatment, it is important to consider the risks to the individual in all these spheres, were the manic episode to continue unabated. If there are persistent risks to health or safety, compulsory admission to hospital may be necessary, for protection and care, and treatment of the manic illness.

Treatment of mania and hypomania

Neuroleptic drugs, lithium, and electro-convulsive therapy (ECT) are all effective in curtailing an episode of mania.

Neuroleptic drugs are usually employed, as their onset of action is rapid, and their calming and sedative effects beneficial. Lithium is reserved for patients who are not behaviourally disordered, because anti-manic effects are delayed until a therapeutic dose is reached. ECT is used only rarely, typically in cases of severe mania resistant to other treatments. Benzodiazepines may be useful as adjuvant treatments, as their sedative effects may permit the use of low doses of neuroleptics, thereby preventing certain adverse effects.

Bipolar disorder is a recurrent illness, and prophylaxis should be considered at an early stage. Lithium salts are still the treatment of first choice for prophylaxis, even though as many as 40 per cent of patients may be unresponsive. Other prophylactic treatments include carbamazepine, sodium valproate, and depot anti-psychotic drugs.

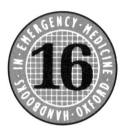

CHAPTER 16

Manipulative behaviour

Introduction

- **Recognition   Management**

Manipulative behaviour is a term often used pejoratively: its use is in describing a variety of situations where the established convention governing the relationship between a health professional and a patient breaks down. This usually occurs when a disparity has emerged between the expectations of the patient and the professional's idea of what is appropriate to provide with the latter feeling pressured and 'manipulated'. Although it is not automatic that the cause lies with the patient, it is hoped that professionals will be able to be more objective in their judgements than patients who are in the emotionally charged position of needing help. It is important to avoid the easy temptation to use the term as a purely pejorative label or a rationale for considering a patient unco-operative and untreatable.

Recognition

Behaviours described as being manipulative may involve one or more of the following:

(1) excessive demands (including use of tactics such as fawning, sycophancy, seduction, coercion, and outright threats of violence);
(2) making the professional feel responsible for the patient's problem;
(3) withholding information;
(4) resistive and subtly unco-operative behaviour;
(5) expressions of resentment;

(6) deceitfulness, outright lying, and fabrication of information.

It is worth remembering, however, that manipulative behaviour may be a manifestation of significant psychiatric disorder. Certainly, hostility or threats of violence in one of previously equable temperament should always arouse suspicion of the presence of mental disorder. Acute confusional states, for example, may be complicated by difficult and unco-operative behaviour, and patients with epilepsy, head injury or other forms of cerebral disease may present in a similar fashion. Patients with schizophrenia often present in crisis, and may resort to manipulation in desperate attempts to obtain help, particularly when their judgement and insight have been affected by illness. Manic patients may feel frustrated and besmirched by doctors who appear dull and wooden, and those in the throes of severe depression may be irritable and unco-operative as a result of brooding, pessimism, and despair. Manipulation and humiliation form much of the currency used by patients with antisocial personalities, who are unable to employ more appropriate techniques such as ventilation, discussion, and compromise. In other forms of personality disorder problems in relationships may habitually lead to excessively demanding behaviour which is seen as manipulative and of course it can be expected to occur in relations with professionals also.

Management

The first step in managing manipulative behaviour is to recognize that it is occurring. It is common to attempt to protect oneself from difficult feelings by humour or intellectualization. Occasionally, doctors may feel angry and act dismissively in a quite uncharacteristic fashion. The feelings aroused by patients should not be regarded as troublesome or challenging, but instead viewed as useful and informative. A moment's reflection on such feelings may provide a useful insight into the nature of the doctor—patient relationship. This in turn allows the doctor to understand the purpose of the patient's behaviour, and possibly also its recognition as a recurring pattern in other relationships. Common responses amongst professional staff to manipulative behaviour need to be recognized. Certain feelings that are uncharacteristic may arise in response to manipulative behaviours on the part of the patient. These may include:

(1) feelings of impotence, and helplessness, combined with uncharacteristic feelings of being asked to take responsibility for a patient;

(2) becoming over-involved with patients and making 'special' efforts on their behalf;

(3) feelings of anger, hostility, and rejection;

(4) actions of a retaliative nature, with attempts to avoid further treatment of the patient.

Fortunately, most professionals are reasonably insightful, and acting on such feelings should become less frequent with accumulating experience.

If a therapeutic relationship is at risk of becoming ruptured, it is important to address this issue by making it available for discussion with the patient. This involves clarifying the limits within which the consultation is being held, in particular what can realistically be expected by the patient to be offered him by the professional.

Conflict can be avoided if both doctor and patient cooperate in solving problems, and observe the limits that are necessary for successful interview and examination. Agreements to disagree on particular problems, whilst attempting to find common ground on other difficulties can be both fruitful and rewarding. It is sometimes helpful to pause for a break during a difficult interview, such 'time out' allowing both parties the opportunity of unwinding and reflection. Following these guidelines may allow the re-establishment of a firm therapeutic relationship, which in turn may allow effective treatment for the patient's legitimate complaint.

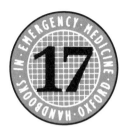

CHAPTER 17

Munchausen syndrome

Introduction

- **Recognition   Immediate management**

The eponym Munchausen syndrome was coined by Asher in 1951 after the widely travelled and dramatically untruthful Baron of this name to describe a chronic disorder involving the presentation of factitious physical symptoms. It was subsequently described as a syndrome of hospital addiction. It entails the deliberate deception of medical services by the presentation of false symptoms and self-induced signs that are suggestive of physical disease, with the resulting offer of medical treatment.

Motivations underlying such behaviour may include any of the following:

(1) material gain in the form of psychoactive drugs of abuse, or free board and lodgings;
(2) avoidance of legal difficulties, through medical sanction;
(3) achieving a caring response from others;
(4) achieving status as the centre of attention.

Munchausen syndrome is often associated with an underlying personality disorder. It may represent an exaggeration of other personality traits of the individual, including an inability to sustain trusting relationships; manipulative, dishonest or sensation-seeking behaviour; and anxiousness or excessive dependence on others. Psychological theorists have seen the choice of the medical field for this essentially maladaptive behaviour as being a consequence of childhood illness or disability leading to prolonged medical treatment and a persisting ambivalence about the caring and powerful aspects of the medical role.

Recognition

Common presentations include abdominal pain, haemorr-
hage, pyrexia of unknown origin, generalized rash, and
chest pain. The diagnosis is generally not apparent at first
presentation, although characteristic features may be noticeable in retrospect:

(1) the patient may be unwilling to provide significant personal details, such as an address or that of the next of
kin;
(2) patients may claim to be in transit, and offer elaborate
and seemingly implausible explanations for their movements (pseudologia fantastica);
(3) the presentation of symptoms may be classical, reflecting
careful rehearsal—leading to retrospective opinions
amongst professionals that symptoms were 'too good to
be true";
(4) the patient may have significant links with the medical
profession, either through family connections, a para-
medical occupation, or as a result of prolonged hospital
stays earlier in life.

If the patient is admitted to hospital, maintenance of symptoms and signs will usually encourage investigation and
treatment, even to the point of invasive and potentially
dangerous procedures. Certain patients, however, will sabo-
tage investigations and avoid attempts to obtain personal
details or verify the medical history. Typically, the nursing
and medical staff become increasingly suspicious, and when
finally challenged the patient responds with angry and re-
sentful statements and a rapid departure from the ward.

Munchausen syndrome was first described in terms of the
factitious presentation of physical complaints. More recently,
other variants have become recognized. Munchausen syndrome may present through a factitious psychiatric disorder,
usually with features of a psychotic illness. Munchausen
syndrome by proxy is increasingly recognized, the protagon-
ist presenting factitious evidence of ill health in dependent
children or elderly persons in their care.

Immediate management

The first objective of management is to confidently exclude a real basis for the presented pathology. This may be impossible without a period of observation in a ward, which to some extent results in the achievement of the patient's aims. Typically, only a short period passes before suspicions are aroused. Sensitive confrontation becomes necessary, which should aim to minimize the trauma to all the involved parties. Medical and nursing staff should state that the deceit has been recognized, and then attempt to provide to help for any practical or remediable problems. It is important to avoid excessive zeal in confrontation, as this may provoke overt aggression on the part of the patient.

Revelation of the deception and avoidance of the expression of understandably negative feelings by staff may allow the elucidation of underlying conflicts and entry into a therapeutic contract. Very often however patients resist such engagement and leave to continue the repetition of their maladaptive relationship with caring professionals elsewhere.

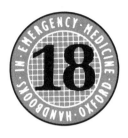

CHAPTER 18

Physically ill patients refusing treatment

Introduction

- **Management**

Trainee psychiatrists often receive enquiries as to whether it is appropriate for physically ill patients to be detained under the Mental Health Act when they refuse treatment. In certain circumstances this is appropriate but only after an exhaustive review of other possible avenues; in the majority of cases, the management of the patient should proceed along rather different lines. Particular problems arise when a patient with an identifiable mental disorder, as well as physical illness, resists necessary medical care and treatment, preferring instead to leave the ward or casualty department and return home.

Management

In many cases, the decision of a physically ill patient to discharge him or herself from a casualty department or a hospital bed is borne out of frustration with delays, and confusion regarding management. Both can result from a failure of communication between staff and patient. In such circumstances, an unhurried, sympathetic, and reasonably detailed clarification of the planned management is sufficient to convince the patient that their best interests are served by remaining in hospital and receiving medical attention.

Most patients who discharge themselves from hospital

are not mentally disordered. Poor decisions based on inadequate information should not necessarily be equated with the disturbance of judgement and insight that is a feature of many psychiatric illnesses. Patients should be allowed to discharge themselves and leave hospital, providing it is clear that they are neither suffering from a mental disorder which is responsible for their decision, nor are likely to come to serious harm as a result of their actions. When a patient has accepted and understood balanced arguments regarding continuing care, and yet persists with the wish to be allowed to leave, the following course is recommended:

1. Decide whether or not you need to inform your superior of the patient's wishes (depending largely on the potential seriousness of failure to receive treatment).

2. Inform the patient that his action is against medical advice, and where indicated intimate the probable risks that this action may involve.

3. Complete a 'discharge against medical advice' form. Typically, this is signed by both the patient and the doctor and is additionally witnessed by a third party, usually a nurse.

4. Record the circumstances and outcome in the case notes.

When a patient chooses to disregard these formalities, and simply absconds from the department the events should be recorded in the medical notes in some detail. When there is significant concern regarding the patient's health (physical or mental) efforts should be made to contact relatives, carers, and the patient's general practitioner.

It is important to remember that 'discharge against medical advice' forms do not absolve medical or nursing staff from the responsibility of assessing a patient properly before allowing him or her to leave hospital.

When it is clear that a patient is not mentally disordered, but there is significant concern regarding risk to life, treatment and care can be provided within the boundaries of Common Law. Doctors and nurses worry about the legitimacy of restraining and treating patients without having obtained consent. In cases of genuine emergency, however, Common Law implies that it is safe to do what is reasonably necessary to save life, or to prevent a serious deterioration in health, without having obtained the consent of a patient. Doctors who act in good faith, in the best interests of a patient, are most unlikely to be criticized during any ensuing legal proceedings.

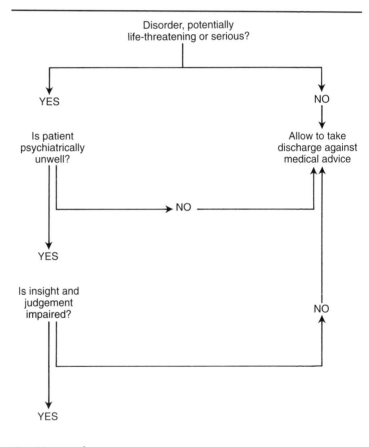

Fig. 1 • Management of the physically ill patient refusing treatment.

In a minority of cases, a patient's decision to refuse treatment and discharge himself from hospital may be determined by mental disorder. This situation occurs most commonly in acutely confused patients, when disorientation, delusions, distressing hallucinations, and agitation may cause a patient to act indecisively or rashly. The management of such patients is described in Chapter 6 on confusion. In other cases, however, a patient's action may be the result of functional psychosis, depression or uncontrollable anxiety. Patients may hold delusions that doctors wish to harm them, or experiment with them; or that they are immune to disease as a result of grandiose delusions. Depressed patients may be inappropriately pessimistic about their condition, or suicidal, or believe that their illness is a deserved punishment.

Where serious physical illness coexists with a known mental disorder, which compromises the willingness to accept treatment for the medical condition, referral to a psychiatrist is necessary. Detention under the provisions of the Mental Health Act may be recommended, but only when the mental disorder is affecting insight and judgement, and the consequences of this is to place the patient's health at significant risk. Compulsory admission does not permit the enforced treatment of medical or surgical problems, only that of the psychiatric disorder. The exception to this is when the physical illness is directly responsible for the patient's psychiatric disorder, for example, an infection or metabolic disorder causing an acute confusional state.

Common Law may have to be invoked for the treatment of physical illnesses when this situation does not apply. When treatment is not urgent, admission to hospital and the institution of psychiatric treatment may result in an improvement in the patient's mental state, to the extent that consent can then be sought and obtained for any necessary medical or surgical intervention.

CHAPTER 19

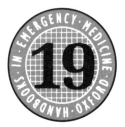

Puerperal psychosis

Introduction

- **Recognition   Immediate management**

Puerperal psychosis is a severe and potentially dangerous mental disorder, which typically arises within the first two weeks of childbirth. Although considerably less common than either 'baby blues' or postnatal depression, puerperal psychosis cannot be considered a rare disorder, there being approximately one case per 500 live deliveries.

Recognition

The clinical picture of puerperal psychosis is quite variable. Approximately 80 per cent of cases are characterized by predominant affective symptoms, similar to those seen in mania or hypomania (see 'Mania and hypomania'). Mixed affective states and depressive psychoses, however, are not uncommon. A minority of patients present with features similar to those seen in acute schizophrenic episodes, but again affective symptoms are usually prominent. Rather less common features of puerperal psychosis include perplexity, poor attention, and disorientation in time and place. True 'organic' psychoses, accompanied by confusional states, arising from puerperal sepsis or other medical complications, are rather less common with improvements in obstetric practice.

Difficulties in the diagnosis of puerperal psychosis stem largely from the non-specific nature of the early symptoms. Anxiety, irritability, tearfulness, and insomnia ('baby blues') are part of normal experience in the first few days of parenthood. Typically, these symptoms peak at around the fifth postpartum day, and then resolve quickly, without the need for intervention other than explanation, understanding, and reassurance. In puerperal psychosis, by contrast, minor affective changes are the harbingers of a florid and disturbing illness which threatens the well-being of mother and baby alike. Delusional beliefs regarding the child may evolve rapidly, hallucinations may be vivid and hard to resist, and behaviour may become seriously disordered. Suicidal thoughts and acts are real risks, as is the possibility of neglect of, or harm to, the baby.

The distinction of late 'blues' from early puerperal psychosis may be difficult, and doctors should always err on the side of caution when making management decisions. It is rather easier to distinguish puerperal psychosis from postnatal depression, which although potentially serious, typically arises several weeks postpartum. Postnatal depression affects some 10–30 per cent of mothers, and is regrettably rather frequently overlooked. The features of this condition are essentially similar to those seen in other forms of depressive illness, although the content of thoughts may be different. Worries regarding oneself, for example, may be replaced by an excessive or inappropriate concern for the health of the child, leading to frequent presentations to family doctors of healthy babies accompanied by anxious and depressed mothers. Postnatal depression is so common, as to lead many authorities to recommend that the 10-item Edinburgh Postnatal Depression Scale (Cox -) be included as a screening instrument within the setting of the routine postnatal follow-up.

Immediate management

Puerperal psychosis is a psychiatric emergency, because the clinical picture is fluctuant and unpredictable, and the hazards of untreated illness are potentially catastrophic. The threshold for admission to hospital should be low, and detention under the provisions of the Mental Health Act used whenever required. Both mother and baby are at risk, and the well-being and safety of significant others may be compromised. Admission to Mother and Baby units is preferable, although patients may be managed effectively in side-rooms of general psychiatric wards, providing vigilant observation by nursing staff is maintained. Such specialist units are ideally placed, when close to obstetric and paediatric wards. With early recognition and prompt treatment, the short-term prognosis for patients with puerperal psychosis is extremely good. Treatment in the short term is primarily physical. Mania-like illnesses, for example, will require treatment with antipsychotic drugs, and depressive psychoses usually resolve following the institution of treatment with electroconvulsive therapy (ECT).

Psychotropic drugs are excreted in breast milk and may cause significant adverse effects (for example, dystonia with antipsychotics) and this therefore demands careful monitoring of dosages. Lithium is contraindicated in breast-feeding mothers due to the significant risk of toxicity in the newborn.

Attention to the interaction of mother and child is important during treatment. Mothers developing ideas that their child is abnormal or deformed are dangerous. Although there is no evidence to suggest that the future well-being of the child may be damaged by the mother's inability to care for a few days, it is important for the mother's recovery to recommence parenting as soon as an improvement begins.

It is probable that many incidences of puerperal psychosis could be prevented. Risk factors for the development of a psychotic illness in the postpartum period include a history of previous puerperal psychosis, a family history of severe mental illness, and a previous personal history of psychosis, particularly manic depressive psychosis. Bipolar patients are at increased risk of developing puerperal psychosis, and should be monitored vigilantly throughout the antenatal and immediate postpartum period. Patients maintained on lithium prior to conception will have been withdrawn from that drug during pregnancy, but it can be re-instituted on the first postpartum day, providing adequate attention is paid to lithium levels, and the mother has no desire to breast-feed her baby.

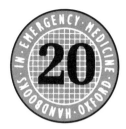

CHAPTER 20

Social crisis

Introduction

- **Homelessness   Acute distress   Relationship crises
  Children at risk**

Social crises are included in a book on the management of psychiatric emergencies because of the importance of the social context in understanding all forms of unusual behaviour. Many of the more extreme forms of social dysfunction may result in behaviour which requires distinguishing from acute psychiatric disorders.

Homelessness

Homelessness is a social problem that is seen to be a major variable in the health, and the access to health care, of an increasing proportion of the population. It should be regarded as resulting from a number of diverse causative factors, both personal, for example, poverty and the breakdown of family relationships, and societal, such as unemployment and the scarcity of low-cost public housing.

The prominence of the mentally ill as a group within the homeless population is a great cause of concern, both to the general public and to those working in the mental health field. Homelessness among this group may be a consequence of the inability of vulnerable patients to sustain contact with psychiatric and other services which have not yet developed effective community alternatives to the traditional mode of care.

Homeless patients are common and visible in casualty departments. This is probably the result of the priority that a homeless person has to give to securing the basic necessities of food, shelter, and clothing. Access to primary health care is less pressing, and can be more difficult as itinerant individuals are not attractive additions to a general practitioner's list. Consequently, homeless patients will inevitably present to casualty departments with problems that are neither accidents nor emergencies.

Management

It is easy to dismiss the presentation of non-acute problems by an unprepossessing individual, since casualty departments are not established to respond to these sorts of difficulties. It is legitimate, however, both to give first aid, and to attempt a first step towards the resolution of the patient's housing predicament.

Obviously, management of any medical condition may be compromised by the lack of accommodation, and the threshold for admission to hospital to guarantee the provision of minimum nutrition, hygiene, and shelter may be lower.

For patients where the medical condition is not so serious as to require hospital admission, there are still contributions that can be made by doctors and other health workers. Casualty departments and hospital-based social workers should maintain an accurate list of local shelters and direct-access hostels, which may provide temporary accommodation with the minimum of formality.

Furthermore, specific groups of patients can claim priority for temporary housing by a local authority on the basis of vulnerability on medical grounds, within the meaning of the 1985 Housing Act. Such patients, which include the elderly, pregnant women, and the mentally ill, can be referred to the local authority homeless persons' unit with evidence, usually in writing, of their vulnerability.

Acute distress

Acutely distressed individuals may naturally seek emergency help in the aftermath of an unprecedented and untoward life event. Typical circumstances include the untimely death of a close relative or friend, exposure to danger or violence, or the witnessing of a major civil disaster. Extreme distress may be characterized by symptoms that are identical to those seen in the major psychiatric disorders. Such features include both the psychological and physical manifestations of anxiety, tearfulness, an apparent unawareness of the surroundings, and disinhibition leading to unrestrained grief and self-castigation.

Management

The first step is the recognition of the provoking events, which are usually reported by the individual, if not by any accompanying persons.

The guiding principle is to avoid excessive 'medicalization' of a problem, whilst at the same time providing the short-term measures which are necessary to reduce gross distress. It may, for example, be appropriate to mobilize support from family and friends, and to provide reassurance that distress will not be prolonged. I may also be appropriate to prescribe hypnotic or anxiolytic drugs, usually benzodiazepines. The reduction of distress arising from threatening or disorientating events is not associated with the development of later psychological symptoms. Naturally, it is important to limit such treatment to short periods.

Family and relationship crises

Doctors often find themselves asked to adjudicate in a dispute arising when the actions of one individual are perceived to impinge on the freedoms of another. Specifically, the doctor may be asked to endorse the invalidation of the viewpoint of an individual, by confirmation of his or her state of (usually mental) ill health.

In this situation it is wise to adopt a cautiously neutral approach, until the presence or absence of mental illness can be clearly established. It may be difficult to judge whether the concern of another family member is appropriate and beneficial where an individual is known to suffer from a mental illness. The relative's view may be coloured by overprotectiveness or infantilization of the ill individual, over-involvement in the affairs of the patient, or through an excessively hostile or critical stance.

Other situations may arise as the result of tensions in marital relationships or other partnerships. Difficulties can occur on a recurrent basis in relationships where one partner is excessively dependent on the other. Problems may arise when excessive demands are made, leading to an unwillingness of the partner to offer continuing support, sometimes to the point of breakdown of the relationship. Psychiatrists regard repeated difficulties of this nature as being relatively frequent in those suffering from personality disorder, but it may also occur in those with other mental illnesses, although on a less recurrent basis.

Management

The first principle is to make explicit one's role as a mediator or facilitator. This may require the temporary suspension of one's role as medical adviser, or even its transfer to a colleague in order to avoid confusing the patient or his or her relatives. The second is to ensure that each party is able to communicate their view clearly and without interruption. The third is to facilitate discussion and to encourage compromise over disputed issues.

Child care proceedings

Social services have a statutory duty to investigate situations where there is reason to believe that a child under the age of 17 may be suffering as a result of parental neglect or abuse. Their interventions in these circumstances are regulated by the Children Act 1989.

Social workers have the duty to assess and monitor situations where children may be at risk. When necessary and in order to fulfil this duty they may seek additional powers from a magistrate. A Child Assessment Order allows access to the family by a social worker, and any other relevant professionals, such as doctors, for the purposes of assessment of the risk within a 7 day period. If significant concern remains the social worker may initiate Care Proceedings during which time a guardian *ad litem* is appointed until one of several outcomes is reached.

1. An Interim Supervision Order allows joint responsibility for the welfare of children to be exercised by parents and social services.
2. A Permanent Care Order allows the removal from parents of children considered at persistent risk and their placement with foster parents or in a children's home.
3. An Emergency Protection Order allows removal of children for up to 8 days in the face of immediate risk to well-being.

Those who suffer from mental illness can be considered inadequate parents if they sustain lengthy periods of dysfunction, or if their illness involves seriously irresponsible or potentially dangerous behaviour. This may be particularly likely if the patient shows an incomplete appreciation of the nature and effects of their illness and the importance of treatment, for example, by declining treatment or ignoring medical advice.

Parents who are subject to such proceedings are likely to respond with considerable suspicion, and at times anger, towards those they see as responsible. This may include professionals, including psychiatrists and other doctors who have presented medical evidence bearing on their ability as parents.

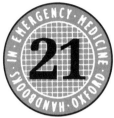

CHAPTER 21

Somatization

Introduction

- **Recognition   Immediate management**

Somatization is a term used to describe the replacement of psychological problems by physical symptoms which are assumed to have an emotional origin. Somatization is more of a process than a syndrome or diagnosis, and involves repeated contact with doctors which is not contingent upon symptoms and fails to be deterred by appropriate reassurance.

By its very nature it therefore results in the presentation of psychologically distressed patients to non-psychiatrists. Somatization is a feature of a number of psychiatric disorders, particularly those that involve disturbances of mood, such as depressive illness. It is also the essential feature of a number of relatively uncommon mental disorders, including primary hypochondiasis, Briquet syndrome, and factitious disorder.

Recognition

Somatization arises from two underlying and interacting factors. An excessive preoccupation with bodily sensations combines with a prevailing fear of physical illness. Normal physiological events, such as tachycardia on exertion or somatic accompaniments of anxiety, come to be regarded as signs of severe physical disease. For example, hyperventilation, commonly occurring in anxiety states, may lead to increased activity in respiratory musculature. If persistent this may lead to tenderness of the chest wall which may then be perceived as evidence of physical ill-health and arouse further anxieties which motivate help-seeking from a professional. Repeated consultations with health professionals result in repetitive examination and inappropriate investigations. Assurance is given but can never be accepted. The frequency of presentation steadily rises, and the doctor–patient relationship gradually deteriorates.

Immediate management

The first task is to conduct sufficient physical examinations and investigations to exclude somatic disease confidently. It is important to strike the right balance between, on the one hand, exhaustive and unnecessary investigations, and on the other, cursory or superficial examinations, which may lead the patient to believe that his or her complaints are not being taken seriously. Difficulties may arise when the presenting complaints are essentially subjective, and not easily verifiable by objective examination.

Certain features are suggestive of somatization:

(1) symptoms and signs which do not conform to recognized clinical entities;
(2) presenting complaints which vary with mood state or social circumstances;
(3) patients who appear to have an excessive degree of conviction that there is no psychological reason for their physical symptoms;
(4) the degree of distress or disability may vary according to whether or not the patient is observed;
(5) a history of repeated consultations for similar symptoms, with increasing investigations although without corresponding reassurance.

Somatization is a common manifestation of certain psychiatric disorders.

(1) **Depressive illness.** Physical symptoms are commonly reported by depressed patients. Loss of appetite and weight, disturbance of sleep, and marked lassitude suggest

the presence of depression. Such 'biological' symptoms are strongly predictive of a good response to antidepressant medication. The diagnosis of depression is supported when depressive cognitions such as self-reproach, hopelessness, and suicidal thoughts are present.

(2) **Anxiety disorders.** Anxiety is characterized by both psychological and somatic symptoms. The latter include musculo-skeletal problems such as headache and stiffness, and autonomic complaints such as palpitation, perceived breathlessness, epigastric discomfort, and diarrhoea. These symptoms may be thought to be indicative of an underlying serious physical illness. Rising concern leads to increasing somatic anxiety, and repeated presentations for reassurance.

(3) **Monosymptomatic hypochondriacal delusional psychosis.** This severe mental illness is characterized by a persistent but relatively circumscribed delusional conviction of the presence of a specific and unremitting physical illness. Affected individuals often show premorbid personality traits of solitariness, suspiciousness, and excessive introspection. The apparent failure of doctors to take these claims seriously results in the presentation of increasingly elaborate 'evidence' of ill health, and with each rebuff the delusion is defended more vigorously.

(4) **Primary hypochondriasis/Briquet syndrome.** A group of patients persist in inappropriate medical consultation in the absence of formally diagnosable mental illness. In this group the persistent maladaptive behaviour can be seen as one manifestation of abnormal personality traits of dependence, attention-seeking, and anxiousness.

It is important to engage the patient through a sympathetic hearing, and not dismiss reported symptoms as being imaginary. Once achieved, the more difficult and time-consuming task of identifying psychological problems can begin. Some patients may accept that they are temporarily experiencing emotional difficulties, and may agree to a referral to a psychiatrist. Others, particularly those with delusional disorders, will be hostile to such a suggestion. A successful referral may result in the definitive treatment of underlying psychiatric disorders, through the use of physical treatments or psychological therapies. Recent success has been claimed for the use of cognitive therapies aimed at correcting the unfounded hypochondriacal assumptions common to these patients.

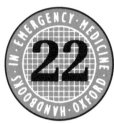

CHAPTER 22

Stupor and mutism

Introduction

- **Recognition Immediate management**

'Stupor' is a term that has rather different meanings to psychiatrists and neurologists. Psychiatrists regard stupor as the syndrome of akinetic mutism, in which patients are silent and immobile, but fully conscious. The undisturbed level of consciousness is verified through the demonstration of purposeful eye movements and the registration of painful stimuli through blinking or grimacing, as well as by clear retrospective accounts of being aware of their surroundings. Neurologists, by contrast, consider stupor to be a disturbance of the level of consciousness.

Recognition

There can be few presentations more dramatic than that of cases of stupor. Typically, the patient lies motionless on a casualty stretcher, unable to speak, yet aware of surrounding activities and attending professionals. When the patient is accompanied by a close informant, the syndrome of stupor can be recognized without great difficulty on the basis of reports of gradually progressive slowing and taciturnity. Often, however, the patient is brought to medical attention by concerned strangers or ambulance staff, when, in the absence of any history the diagnosis of stupor should be made only after thorough investigation.

The list of possible causes of stupor is extensive, encompassing psychiatric and neurological conditions.

(1) **Psychiatric causes.** Stupor is an uncommon presentation of a number of common illnesses, including

dementia, schizophrenia, and depression. Manic stupor is seen only rarely, and can usually only be diagnosed in retrospect, when the previously mute patient becomes able to describe a sense of exhaustion, accompanied by ecstasy and racing thoughts. Hysterical stupor should be diagnosed with great caution, only after all other causes have been excluded, and when there is evidence of both primary and secondary gain from such a state.

(2) **Neurological causes.** The syndrome of akinetic mutism, with disturbance of the level of consciousness, can be produced by a variety of neurological disorders. Epilepsy may be a factor, stupor occurring in both ictal and post-ictal states. Encephalitis is an uncommon cause, as are lesions of the frontal and temporal lobes, or of the posterior diencephalon. Other neurological causes include Parkinson's disease, and neuroleptic drug overdosage.

(3) **Other medical causes.** The syndrome of stupor may be produced by a disparate range of conditions, including hepatic encephalopathy, hypoglycaemia, hypergly-caemia, and uraemia.

'Organic' factors probably account for around 20 per cent of cases of stupor. Without corroborative information, it is extremely difficult to distinguish organic from psychiatric causes of stupor, and patients in such states should always be regarded as medical emergencies, unless previous presentations have consistently been found to have a psychogenic cause. Clinical features which suggest a neurological cause include a relatively sudden onset, and evidence of abnormality on neurological examination. Alterations in the level of consciousness are suggestive of neurological causes, as is a progressive course with increasing obtundity and emerging neurological signs.

In patients with stupor caused by psychiatric illness, there is often a history of previous similar presentations, and a recent history of stressful life events. Examination in such patients may reveal a blissfully serene appearance, tearfulness, or frequent blinking, the latter suggesting the presence of auditory hallucinations. Occasionally, stupor due to schizophrenia may be associated with catatonic phenomena such as waxy flexibility and negativism.

Immediate management

Stupor is a syndrome, not a diagnosis. Underlying causes should always be sought in a rigorous fashion. This process involves seeking information from other sources, including informants and medical records. The patient should be admitted to hospital, which may require implementation of the Mental Health Act. Nursing observation should be especially vigilant, as catatonic stupor can suddenly change to a state of excitement, with consequent risks to the patient, others, and property. It is essential to perform a physical examination and as much examination of the mental state as is feasible. Rehydration and parenteral feeding may be required when the syndrome has persisted more than a few hours. Investigations should include estimations of blood glucose, and of urea and electrolytes. Further investigations might include a CT scan of the head and electroencephalography. In psychiatric causes of stupor, the EEG is typically that seen in the normal waking state, or characterized by only non-specific changes. In organic causes, the EEG is more likely to be abnormal, with evidence either of focal abnormality, or of generalized diffuse slowing.

Treatment of the patient in stupor should only be instituted once the cause is clear. Benzodiazepine anxiolytics, when prescribed in low dosage, may produce beneficial effects by reducing muscle tone and diminishing arousal, to the extent that discussion with the patient becomes possible. Neuroleptic drugs may be appropriate in cases of stupor due to schizophrenia or mania, and electroconvulsive therapy (ECT) may produce dramatic effects in those with severe depression.

PART 3

Procedures

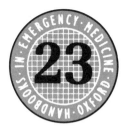

CHAPTER 23

Emergency use of psychotropic drugs

Introduction

- **Antipsychotic drugs—indications, and mode of use**
  Hypnotic anxiolytics—indications, and mode of use

Most drug treatments used in psychiatric practice are prescribed only after a careful and complete assessment, and in standard courses of relatively fixed dosage and duration. For example, antidepressant drugs are typically given over a period of four to six weeks to ameliorate symptoms in the acute phase of major depression. It is therefore not usually appropriate to plan drug treatment for psychiatric disorders in the middle of an emergency presentation occasioned by a crisis of one sort or another. Similarly, consideration of the use of psychotropic drugs in the continuation (where symptoms have responded but the underlying disease is conceptualized to remain), and in the prophylactic phase of treatment (to avoid recurrence of a relapsing disorder) in an emergency is inappropriate.

There are occasions, however, when drugs are justifiably used as the most rapid means of resolution of a tense situation. This most commonly occurs when a distressed and agitated patient is unable to be contained by the physical presence and reassurance of professionals and others, and where behaviour remains unpredictable. Drugs most useful in these situations are antipsychotic and sedative drugs.

Antipsychotic drugs

Also known collectively as neuroleptics, the antipsychotic drugs include a group of pharmacologically disparate agents, all sharing the effect of reducing the intensity of pathological false beliefs and perceptions. This action is thought to result from the antagonism of dopamine receptor activity in specific CNS pathways, particularly the mesolimbic-cortical system. This is consistent with, and indeed is an important piece of evidence supporting the so-called 'dopamine hypothesis' of schizophrenia. Of equal importance is the recent evidence that drugs such as clozapine, which posse only modest dopamine antagonist effects are nevertheless effective antipsychotic agents, which suggests that modification of other receptors (such as those responsive to serotonin), is also important.

Most antipsychotic agents are non-selective in their activity, with effects across a range of important receptors. Significant activities in addition to dopamine blockade include:

(1) antihistaminergic activity, associated with sedative effects;
(2) anticholinergic activity, associated with autonomic effects such as tremor, tachycardia, and constipation;
(3) antiadrenergic actions, associated with postural hypotension.

In addition, dopamine blockade in the nigro-striatal tracts is implicated in the aetiology of extra-pyramidal adverse effects.

Indications for acute use

(1) psychotic symptoms in acute functional and organic psychosis;
(2) agitation and over-activity;
(3) anxiety;
(4) sedation.

Mode of use

1. **Selection of agent.** Antipsychotics are often described as having either high or low potency. 'High potency' agents (such as the buryrophenone and benzamide groups) have relatively more specificity for dopaminergic activity, and correspondingly greater molar efficacy than less selective 'low potency' agents (such as the phenothiazine group).

'Low potency' drugs can also be anticipated to produce fewer extra-pyramidal symptoms, such as tremor,
rigidity, and dystonia, although the inherent anticholinergic activity of some of these drugs is an additional
factor. In general, a 'high potency' drug is preferable
where psychosis is severe and behaviour disturbed or
unpredictable, with 'low potency' drugs reserved for
patients at higher risk of extra-pyramidal syndromes,
such as the elderly and the organically impaired. All
agents have the effect of reducing motor overactivity, but
those with significant sedative effects, such as the pheno-
thiazines, are more quieting.

2. **Mode of administration.** Antipsychotic agents are available for oral (tablet, slow-release capsules, and liquid)
and parenteral (intramuscular and intravenous) administration. In acute use, parenteral preparations should be
reserved for patients who are both unco-operative
through a lack of insight and where failure of compliance
is likely to lead to dangerous and irresponsible behaviour. Parenteral treatment without consent can be
given under Common Law, if judged necessary to avert
serious injury, but repeated use should be legitimized
through the use of the Mental Health Act. Parenteral use,
particularly by the intravenous route, can be associated
with hypotension and respiratory depression, as well as
with an increased risk of acute dystonias, probably as a
result of higher peak plasma levels of the drug occurring
through the avoidance of first-pass hepatic metabolism.

3. **Dose titration.** Although parameters such as age, sex, and
body mass are approximate guides to dosage, the wide
variation amongst individuals in the ability to metabolize
antipsychotic drugs results in a certain amount of 'trial
and error' when estimating dose regimens. Since the development of antipsychotic effects is delayed for several
days, psychiatrists tend to gauge the achievement of an
effective dosage by the emergence of more immediate if
subtle extra-pyramidal effects. At this point, the dose can
be reduced to one which produces fewer extra-pyramidal
effects, but which retains antipsychotic efficacy.

Acute adverse effects

1. **Acute dystonic reactions.** Dramatic spasms of skeletal muscles, typically involving central musculature such as the oro-bucco-lingual, cervical or extra-ocular groups, which are alarming for patients and require immediate administration of anticholinergic agents, sometimes parenterally.

2. **Akathisia.** An uncomfortable subjective feeling of motor restlessness, often leading to relentless pacing behaviour, which responds best to a reduction in antipsychotic dosage.

3. **Sedation.** This may be a desirable effect in an overactive or disinhibited patient, but in the longer term is associated with morbidity and non-compliance.

4. **Postural hypotension.**

5. **Neuroleptic malignant syndrome.** This is a disputed and as yet incompletely understood condition, characterized by muscular rigidity, alteration of conscious level, autonomic instability including hyperpyrexia, and elevation of serum levels of the muscle enzyme, creatinine phosphokinase (CPK). It is a serious and potentially life-threatening condition, which requires immediate withdrawal of antipsychotic agents and supportive medical treatment.

Interactions

Combination of antipsychotic agents with other sedative drugs (including alcohol) may result in the potentiation of any sedative effects. Drugs which compete for hepatic hydroxylation (for example, tricyclic antidepressants) or plasma protein binding sites will also potentiate effects.

Hypnotic anxiolytics

Barbiturates have now been superseded by the benzodiazepines, which include a range of drugs with similar pharmacological activity, but differing mainly in their duration of activity. Benzodiazepines combine the following clinical actions:

(1) sedation;
(2) reduction in psychic (and somatic) anxiety;
(3) anticonvulsant action;
(4) muscle relaxation.

Indications for use

(1) anxiety;
(2) insomnia;
(3) substitution for drugs which have induced chemical dependency;
(4) muscle relaxation;
(5) epilepsy.

Mode of use

Benzodiazepines may be used in short-term and symptomatic treatment, often in an adjunctive role to more specific agents, for example, antidepressants and antipsychotic drugs. Agents with longer half-lives should be selected unless only a brief duration of hypnotic activity is desired, or the patient complains of continued and excessive sedation. Doses should be maintained as low as possible, and use limited to periods of under two weeks, and if possible on intermittent days to minimize the risk of dependence. Parenteral administration is occasionally useful to quieten agitated and overexcited patients, although it is claimed that benzodiazepines may 'release' aggression.

Adverse effects

(1) induction of physical dependence;
(2) prolonged sedation if combined with alcohol;
(3) release of aggression.

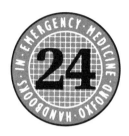

CHAPTER 24

Emergency use of the Mental Health Act

Introduction

- **Use of the Act**   **Details of the Sections**

The purpose of the Mental Health Act (1983), and its equivalent legislation in Scotland and Northern Ireland (see Appendix 1), is to regulate the use of involuntary forms of psychiatric intervention and treatment. As well as defining the rights of the patient, it also serves to legitimize the proper actions of health professionals who may need to override the wishes of an individual whose insight or judgement is impaired.

The Act defines mental illness, subnormality, severe subnormality, and psychopathic disorder. It also stipulates broad conditions governing the circumstances where the Act can be employed: to avoid risk of harm to the health and safety of the patient or to protect other persons.

The Act is a legal document divided into several parts, covering areas such as consent to treatment, admission for assessment, and admission for treatment. Each part is divided into sections which describe the detailed provisions and guidelines. The Mental Health Act Commission (MHAC) is an independent regulatory body with the status of a Special Health Authority, and the duty to interpret the Act. It does so through tribunals in individual cases, through the inspection of hospitals, and by publishing regularly updated editions of the Code of Practice.

Use of the Act

Several professional groups have clearly defined roles in the implementation of the Act. Doctors have a role in not only the diagnosis of mental disorder, but also in the judgement of a patient's ability to recognize this disorder, and to follow medical advice. Additionally, doctors are obliged to consider the likely consequences of failure to follow such advice. If the doctor believes the patient is unreliable and the consequences are sufficiently serious, a written recommendation for admission under a Section may be given to an approved social worker (ASW) who considers whether to accept the application. The ASW is approved by the Secretary of State for Health as having received a specialist training in the mental health field.

Any registered medical practitioner may make a recommendation, including general practitioners and most grades of hospital doctor, including casualty officers but not preregistration house officers. It is desirable, however, to procure recommendations from the most experienced practitioner available within the hospital hierarchy, and from a practitioner with prior knowledge of the patient. It is also mandatory that no two recommendations are from doctors employed by the same health authority. Powers to rescind the Section are restricted to the Responsible Medical Officer (RMO) of the hospital, legally defined as the consultant responsible for the care of the patient.

The ASW has the duty of consulting with the patient's next of kin as well as with the patient, and may accept or decline the medical recommendation(s). If accepted, the patient becomes immediately subject to the provisions of the Section, and the receipt of papers by the hospital managers (or their deputies out of hours, in the form of the senior nursing officer) formalizes admission to hospital. If the recommendations are declined, the professionals in consultation have a duty to jointly plan an alternative course of informal treatment.

Those responsible for the assessment or treatment of patients subject to the Act may call upon the police for assistance. This includes the use of physical force where necessary. It also allows the police to return to hospital a patient who has absconded without medical leave.

The Act draws no legal distinction between wards designated as psychiatric or general. It is therefore appropriate, for example, to use the Act to ensure the admission of a patient to a medical or surgical ward, as well as to a psychiatric ward, providing the purpose is to allow assessment or treatment of their mental as opposed to physical state. The only exception to this is the allowance of treatment of a physical condition which is directly implicated in the mental disorder (for example, treating the organic cause of an acute confusional state).

For the purposes of the Act, the Accident and Emergency department is not considered to be part of the hospital establishment, unlike an in-patient wards, but rather as a place to which the public have a right of access. It is therefore illegal to consider a patient voluntarily attending the Accident and Emergency department as agreeing to voluntary treatment or admission to hospital, but conversely he or she could be considered liable to Section 136 (see below).

All Sections of the Act extend for periods of time, up to a stated maximum. It is within the powers of the RMO (being the consultant in whose care the patient remains), to rescind the Section in writing, at any time before this period has elapsed, thereby allowing the patient to become an informal patient. It is also possible for the nearest relative of the patient to discharge a patient from a Section by giving 72 hours written notice to the hospital managers. However, the RMO has the option to override this mandate and uphold the Section during this 72-hour period. Patients may also be discharged from Sections by the decisions of the hospital managers or Mental Health Review Tribunals (MHRT) to which patients have statutory rights of appeal.

Details of the Sections

Part 2 of the Act deals with compulsory admission for assessment which is most relevant to the management of emergency psychiatric disorder.

Section 2 is most commonly used for assessment purposes. It allows the detention of a patient in hospital (or registered nursing home) for up to 28 days for assessment and treatment. It requires joint or separate recommendations from two doctors to be accepted by an approved social worker (ASW).

Section 4 is used for emergency admission to hospital, on the recommendation of only one doctor, when any delay in securing a second recommendation could allow a dangerous situation to develop. Its duration is restricted to 72 hours, during which time the acceptance of a second medical recommendation results in its conversion to Section 2.

Neither Sections 2 nor 4 sanction repeated or planned treatment of a patient against his or her will; emergency treatment may, however, be given. Only treatment directed at the mental disorder is included in the Act.

Section 5(2) allows a patient who has already agreed to informal admission to be detained against his or her will, on the receipt by the hospital managers of one medical recommendation from the responsible medical officer, or his named deputy (in practice, a named junior doctor on a published hospital rota). The duration of up to 72 hours is designed to allow further assessment with a view to recommendation of Section 2 (for more prolonged in-patient assessment) or 3 (for treatment).

Section 136 allows a police officer to bring to a 'place of safety' any individual who is in a place 'to which the public have access' whose behaviour leads the officer to believe that he or she is mentally disordered and causing a public disturbance. The purpose is to secure assessment by both a medical practitioner and an ASW, with a view to further assessment or treatment (on a voluntary or compulsory basis). It allows the police officer to detain an individual for up to 72 hours whilst this assessment proceeds. 'Places of safety' include police stations and psychiatric wards, but not Accident and Emergency departments. Section 136 automatically expires when assessment is completed by a doctor and ASW, whether or not it leads to acceptance of a further Section, thereby allowing continuing management on a formal or informal basis.

Although rarely appropriate to the emergency situation (except in the case where the patient is well known to the service), Section 3 of the Act allows compulsory admission of a patient to hospital for the purpose of treatment of a mental disorder for a period of up to six months on the acceptance of two medical recommendations by an approved social worker.

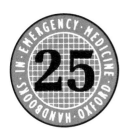

CHAPTER 25

Liaison with psychiatric services

Introduction

- **Range of psychiatric services**

Many of the clinical presentations discussed in this book will benefit from the involvement of the psychiatric services; in some cases, their involvement will be mandatary. This chapter is a guide to referrers to enable them to use specialist psychiatric services effectively.

The way in which psychiatric services are organized, and the methods with which they operate, is currently the subject of much debate. Marked differences exist between services, and it is important that referring agents establish the exact mode of local service delivery. Until 50 years ago, psychiatric services, with the exception of psychotherapy, marriage guidance, and child guidance clinics, were essentially institutional. The care of those requiring psychiatric treatment generally involved admission to a mental hospital. Some treatment was provided by psychiatrists operating from outpatient clinics attached to general hospitals, but for most serious illnesses the main site of treatment was in the mental hospital.

For a range of reasons (including changes in the attitude of society, advances in psychological and physical treatments, and financial considerations) this model of care has been superseded by a different type of service that attempts to provide treatment in a setting which is as least institutional as possible. In practice, this results in patients with chronic mental illness living with families or in group homes, receiving a range of continuing and rehabilitative treatments on a community or out-patient clinic basis. In-patient treatment is increasingly reserved for those patients whose unreliable behaviour temporarily precludes their continuing residence in the community.

The first result of these changes was the appearance of psychiatric units within the district general hospital. These units were geared to responding to patients referred by other services within the hospital, particularly the Accident and Emergency department, which in many cases became the main conduit through which urgent cases presented. General practitioners were served by out-patient clinics and by the availability of day hospitals and centres.

Since these changes, the locus of service delivery has shifted further into the community. Psychiatrists and other mental health professionals now spend a significant amount of time in liaison with agencies scattered throughout a local catchment area, and much clinical work is performed in patients' homes.

Psychiatric services are delivered by multi-disciplinary teams, which include psychiatrists, community psychiatric nurses, social workers, occupational therapists, and clinical psychologists. This diversity reflects the multi-factorial aetiology of most psychiatric disorders, and the range of treatments and interventions which are available for a given clinical problem. The team is involved in the care of patients both in the hospital and in the community, thereby reducing the artificial gap between these two aspects of the service. Generally, there is one point of contact for referrers to the service (administrator during office hours and on-call doctor at other times), but this allows access to all the disciplines without the need for re-referral within the service.

Most teams work to an eclectic model, which acknowledges the biological, psychological, and social aspects of a clinical problem, although some teams employ a more restricted and doctrinaire view of mental illness. Most will embrace a philosophy of assertive outreach and early intervention, the systematic processing of referrals, and a wide network of liaison with community agencies, including general practitioners. Unlike many medical services, psychiatric teams are responsible for defined catchment areas. Only those patients living within the area are eligible to be treated by the service. Emergency referrals will be offered immediate treatment when necessary, but continuing care will be arranged with the relevant local service. This arrangement has arisen from the need for joint social service and health service input, which is difficult to co-ordinate when a multiplicity of adjoining services are involved. The existing arrangement may change as a result of current NHS reorganization, which creates competing providers for services.

The range of psychiatric services

When referring to psychiatric services, it is worth specifying what is required, and the degree of urgency. It should also be clear whether medical responsibility is retained by the referring doctor, or whether the expectation is for this to be assumed by the psychiatrist. Specialist services can supply some or all of the following interventions on an urgent basis

(1) advice regarding diagnosis, risk of suicidal behaviour or aggression, and the optimal choice of treatment;
(2) access to a level of care and treatment that is unavailable outside the specialist service;
(3) assessment with a view to recommendation and application for admission to hospital under a Section of the Mental Health Act;
(4) continuation of treatment and monitoring of response by individuals with appropriate expertise;
(5) rehabilitative care for those with enduring impairments, disabilities, and handicaps.

For services which are predominantly hospital based, emergency assessments are usually the responsibility of a trainee psychiatrist, with support from senior staff on-call. Social workers are often involved in urgent referrals, reflecting their statutory role in formal Mental Health Act assessments. Certain hospitals have walk-in clinics for self-referrals or cases referred by other professionals, manned by psychiatrists and psychiatric nurses. Management options include admission to hospital on a voluntary or compulsory basis, or the initiation of treatment to be continued in the out-patient clinic or by the general practitioner. For community-based services, the response time is liable to be longer, although most teams are able to guarantee a response within 24 hours for urgent cases. Some teams provide an out-of-hours service, enabling the patient to be seen more quickly. The referring doctor may be expected to remain involved in the treatment of the patient, perhaps through starting a prescription, and retaining medical responsibility. Community-based teams may assess patients at home, or in other settings such as health centres, hostels, and group homes.

APPENDIX 1

Mental Health Legislation in Scotland and Northern Ireland

The Mental Health Act (1983) applies only in England and Wales. Elsewhere in the United Kingdom separate legislation exists to regulate the treatment of mental illness, which, whilst following similar principles, differs in detail. Some of the more important provisions relevant to emergency work are considered below.

The Mental Health Act (Scotland) 1984

Admission for assessment

Section 24 allows admission to hospital for assessment in the case of emergency for up to 72 hours on the recommendation of a single medical practitioner and the agreement of either the nearest relative or a mental health officer (a social worker with training in mental health work).

Section 26 allows admission for up to 28 days for assessment and treatment under the same requirements.

Holding powers

Detention of informally admitted in-patients is governed by Section 25 and allows detention for 72 hours on the recommendation of the RMO or nominated deputy. Section 25(4) allows detention for a period of 2 hours on the recommendation of a nurse.

Admission for treatment

Compulsory treatment is regulated by section 18 and requires an application to a sheriff by the mental health officer or nearest relative.

Police powers with regard to the mentally disordered

Section 118 allows a police officer to take to a place of safety for a period of up to 72 hours for the purposes of assessment by a doctor and mental health officer an individual considered to be mentally disordered found in a place to which the public have access.

Mental Health (Northern Ireland) Order (1986)

Admission for assessment

The mechanism for assessment differs significantly, and is regulated by articles 4 and 6 of the Order. A patient can be considered for admission for up to 14 days in the first instance. This requires an application either by a single medical practitioner (article 6) or by the nearest relative or an approved social worker (article 4) to the hospital. This application can be accepted by a doctor on the staff of the receiving hospital on an interim basis and continues to allow detention for a further period. This period is up to 7 days when examination by the RMO has occurred, and for only 48 hours after examination by a less senior doctor (see article 9(1) below).

At the end of either of these periods the admission for assessment can be extended for a further seven days by the RMO. Alternatively, and at any other time during this process, the patient can be regraded to informal status or accepted for compulsory treatment as an inpatient under article 12 (see below).

If the RMO does not examine the patient during this procedure a recommendation by a junior doctor allows detention for 48 hours only under article 9(1).

Holding powers

Article 7 allows detention of an informally admitted patient for up to 48 hours upon receipt of a single medical recommendation, and article 7(3) for 6 hours on receipt of a nursing recommendation.

Admission for treatment

Article 12 governs admission for purposes of treatment and follows the recommendation of the RMO relating to patients already detained under articles 4 or 6.

Police powers with regard to the mentally disordered

Article 130 allows a police officer to detain for up to 48 hours to allow assessment by an ASW and doctor a person considered to be mentally disordered who is found in a place to which the public have access.

Suggested further reading

General

Gelder, Gath, and Mayou (1989). *Oxford textbook of psychiatry.* Oxford University Press.

Hill, Murray and Thorley (1986). *Essentials of post-graduate psychiatry.* Academic Press.

Hawton and Cowen (1990). *Dilemmas and difficulties in the management of psychiatric patients.* Oxford University Press.

Cox, Holden, and Sagovsky (1987). Detection of post-natal depression: development of the 10-item Edinburgh Post-natal Depression Scale. *British Journal of Psychiatry*, **150**, 782–8.

Wallace and Haines (1985). Use of a questionnaire in general practice to increase the recognition of problem drinkers. *British Medical Journal*, 290, 212–14. (CAGE questionnaire).

Classification and diagnosis

World Health Organization (1992). *The ICD-10 classification of mental and behavioural disorders; clinical descriptions and diagnostic guidelines.* WHO.

American Psychiatric Association (1994). *Diagnostic and statistical manual* (4th edn) (DSM IV). APA,

Organic psychiatry

Lishman (1987). *Organic psychiatry.* Blackwell.

Descriptive psychopathology

Sims (1988). *Symptoms in the mind.* Bailziere Tindall.

Drug treatment

Cookson, Cramer, and Heine (1993). *The use of drugs in psychiatry.* Wright.

Mental Health Act

Jones (1991). *Mental Health Act manual.* Sweet and Maxwell.

Index